Clinical Anaesthesia
Lecture Notes

To a wonderful wife and marvellous, uncomplaining mother.

Clinical Anaesthesia
Lecture Notes

Carl Gwinnutt

MB BS MRCS LRCP FRCA
Formerly Consultant Anaesthetist
Salford Royal Hospital NHS Foundation Trust
Honorary Clinical Lecturer in Anaesthesia
University of Manchester, UK

Matthew Gwinnutt

MB ChB (Hons)
Core Trainee in Anaesthesia
Mersey Deanery
Liverpool, UK

Fourth Edition

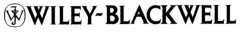

A John Wiley & Sons, Ltd., Publication

Library of Congress Cataloging-in-Publication Data

Lecture notes. Clinical anaesthesia / Carl Gwinnutt, Matthew Gwinnutt. – 4th ed.
    p. ; cm.
  Clinical anaesthesia
  Includes bibliographical references and index.
  ISBN 978-0-470-65892-5 (pbk. : alk. paper)
  I. Gwinnutt, Matthew.   II. Title.   III. Title: Clinical anaesthesia.
  [DNLM: 1.   Anesthesia. 2.   Anesthetics. WO 200]
  617.9′6–dc23

                                                                    2012007478

A catalogue record for this book is available from the British Library.

Cover image: Juan Herrera, iStock Photo
Cover design: Grounded design

Wiley also publishes its books in a variety of electronic formats. Some content that appears in print may not be available in electronic books.

Set in 8.5/11pt, Utopia-Regular by Thomson Digital, Noida, India.
Printed and bound in Malaysia by Vivar Printing Sdn Bhd

2   2013

Contents

List of contributors, vi

Preface, vii

Acknowledgements, viii

List of abbreviations, ix

1　Anaesthetic assessment and preparation for surgery, 1

2　Anaesthetic equipment and monitoring, 18

3　Drugs and fluids used during anaesthesia, 39

4　The practice of general anaesthesia, 58

5　Local and regional anaesthesia, 79

6　Special circumstances, 88

7　Post-anaesthesia care, 100

8　The acutely ill adult patient on the ward, 121

　　Section 1: Recognition and assessment, 121

　　Section 2: Management of common emergencies, 131

Answers to short-answer questions, 159

Answers to true/false questions, 171

Index, 177

Contributor

Anthony McCluskey
Consultant in Anaesthesia and Critical Care
Stockport NHS Foundation Trust
Stepping Hill Hospital
Stockport, UK

Preface

It is now over 15 years since I embarked upon the first edition of this book, and with each subsequent edition I have tried to respond to the demands of the readers and the changes within the specialty of anaesthesia itself. In recent years the anaesthetist's role has expanded dramatically from simply 'providing the conditions under which surgery can be performed safely' and now involves contact with the majority of patients admitted to hospital. This includes playing a major role in preoperative assessment and postoperative care, acute and chronic pain management, as well as the recognition, resuscitation and management of the critically ill. This edition sees many changes to reflect this.

The first major change to this edition is the loss of the chapter giving an overview of critical care. During my career in anaesthesia I have been privileged to see this specialty grow from the efforts of groups of enthusiasts to its recent formal recognition and the formation of the Faculty of Intensive Care Medicine within the Royal College of Anaesthestists. Consequently, I would encourage students to turn to the many excellent texts available on this fascinating and evolving specialty.

The next change in this edition is a reorganization of the way anaesthesia is presented. Firstly, information on equipment, monitoring and the drugs and fluids you will see anaesthetists use in their everyday practice. This is followed by an overview of 'giving an anaesthetic', which describes the processes and procedures used to ensure the patient's safety.

Also included is a small chapter covering some of the specialist branches of anaesthesia that students may encounter; it has not been possible to cover every one and I hope those whose specialties are not included will understand.

Trainees from many specialties now work as part of the 'Hospital at Night' team, and one of their roles is to respond to requests for help with acutely ill patients that they may not be familiar with. Following on from the success of the chapter in the previous edition on the recognition and management of the acutely ill patient on the ward, this has now been expanded into two sections; the first on recognition and assessment of these challenging patients, followed by advice on how initially to manage commonly encountered problems.

But perhaps the greatest change for this edition is that I now welcome my son, as he embarks on a career in anaesthesia, as co-author. He has provided a fresh insight into the specialty as seen by an anaesthetist in training, and is more aware of what medical students need to know, rather than what I think they ought to know. He has worked tirelessly on the manuscript and provided new photographic illustrations; for that I owe him enormously – thank you!

I close by reiterating what I said at the end of the preface of the previous edition, but this time the message comes from both of us; we hope you enjoy this book, but even more we hope it helps you care for your patients. If it has, tell your friends; if it hasn't, tell us why and we'll try to ensure that the next edition is even better!

Acknowledgments

I would like to thank Intersurgical for Figures 2.3 and 2.5, Aircraft Medical for Figure 2.7(d), and Tanya Lachlan, Deltex Medical for Figures 2.18 and 2.19. Figure 2.10 is from McGuire and Younger, 2010 (see useful information section in Chapter 2), with permission of Oxford University Press on behalf of the British Journal of Anaesthesia.

Figures 8.6, 8.7, 8.8 and 8.9 are reproduced with kind permission from Michael Scott and the Resuscitation Council (UK).

Figure 4.12 is reproduced with permission of Dr. P. Ross and I am grateful to Dr J. Corcoran for his help and advice with transversus abdominis plane blocks and Figure 5.2.

Thanks are due to the Difficult Airway Society for Figure 6.3 and the National Tracheostomy Safety Project for Figures 8.1 and 8.2.

I would also like to express my sincere gratitude to Dr Richard Morgan, Professor Gary Smith and Dr Jas Soar for their contributions to the previous edition, some of which by necessity have been included in this edition.

Abbreviations

AAGBI	Association of Anaesthetists of Great Britain and Ireland	DBP	diastolic blood pressure
		DBS	double-burst simulation
ABG	arterial blood gas	DNAR	do not attempt resuscitation
ACE-I	angiotensin converting enzyme inhibitors	DS	degrees of substitution
ACS	acute coronary syndrome	DVT	deep vein thrombosis
ADH	antidiuretic hormone	ECF	extracellular fluid
AKI	acute kidney injury	ECG	electrocardiograph
ALS	advanced life support	EEG	electroencephalograph
AMI	acute myocardial infarction	EMLA	eutectic mixture of local anaesthetic
ANTT	antiseptic no-touch technique	ENT	ear, nose, and throat
ARDS	acute respiratory distress syndrome	ETT	exercise tolerance test
ASA	American Society of Anesthesiologists	EWS	early warning score
AT	anaerobic threshold	FAST	focused assessment with sonography in trauma
ATN	acute tubular necrosis		
BIS	bispectral index	FBC	full blood count
BMI	body mass index	FEV_1	forced expiratory volume in 1 second
BNF	British National Formulary	FFP	fresh frozen plasma
BiPAP	bilevel positive airway pressure	FiO_2	fractional inspired oxygen concentration
BP	blood pressure	FRC	functional residual capacity
BTS	British Thoracic Society	FVC	forced vital capacity
CAP	community-acquired pneumonia	GCS	Glasgow Coma Scale
CCU	coronary care unit	GFR	glomerular filtration rate
CEPOD	Confidential Enquiry into Perioperative Death	GI	gastrointestinal
		GIFTASUP	guidelines on IV fluid therapy for adult surgical patients
CNS	central nervous system		
CO_2	carbon dioxide	GTN	glyceryl trinitrate
COPD	chronic obstructive pulmonary disease	HAFOE	high airflow oxygen enrichment
COX	cyclo-oxygenase enzyme	HAP	hospital acquired pneumonia
CPAP	continuous positive airway pressure	Hb	haemoglobin
CPR	cardiopulmonary resuscitation	HbA1c	glycosylated haemoglobin
CPX	cardiopulmonary exercise	HDU	high dependency unit
CRP	c-reactive protein	HIV	human immunodeficiency virus
CRT	capillary refill time	HR	heart rate
CSF	cerebrospinal fluid	HRT	hormone replacement therapy
CT	computerised tomography	5-HT	5-hydroxytryptamine
CTPA	computerised tomography pulmonary angiography	HTLV	human T-cell lymphotrophic virus
		ICF	intracellular fluid
CVC	central venous catheter	ICP	intracranial pressure
CVP	central venous pressure	I:E ratio	inspiratory:expiratory ratio
CVS	cardiovascular system	ILM	intubating LMA
CXR	chest X-ray	INR	international normalized ratio
DAS	Difficult Airway Society	IPPV	intermittent positive pressure ventilation

IR	immediate release		PACU	post-anaesthesia care unit
IV	intravenous		PCA	patient-controlled anaesthesia
IVC	inferior vena cava		PCI	percutaneous coronary intervention
IVRA	intravenous regional anaesthesia		PCV	pressure-controlled ventilation
JVP	jugular venous pressure		PE	pulmonary embolism
K^+	potassium ions		PEA	pulseless electrical activity
kPa	kilopascals		PEEP	positive end expiratory pressure
LBBB	left bundle branch block		PEFR	peak expiratory flow rate
LED	light-emitting diode		PMGV	piped medical gas and vacuum system
LFT	liver function test		PaO_2	arterial partial pressure of oxygen
LMA	laryngeal mask airway		POCT	point of care testing
LP	lumbar puncture		PONV	postoperative nausea and vomiting
LSD	lysergic acid diethylamide		psi	pounds per square inch
MAC	minimum alveolar concentration		PT	prothrombin time
MAP	mean arterial pressure		ROSC	return of spontaneous circulation
MET	metabolic equivalent		RRT	renal replacement therapy
MH	malignant hyperpyrexia		RSI	rapid-sequence induction
MI	myocardial infarction		SBP	systolic blood pressure
MR	modified release		SpO_2	peripheral oxygen saturation
MRI	magnetic resonance imaging		STEMI	ST-segment elevation myocardial infarction
Na^+	sodium ions			
NCEPOD	National Confidential Enquiry into Patient Outcome and Death		SVC	superior vena cava
			TAP	transversus abdominis plane
NIBP	non-invasive blood pressure		TCI	target-controlled infusion
NICE	National Institute for Health and Clinical Excellence		TIVA	total intravenous anaesthesia
			TOF	train-of-four
N_2O	nitrous oxide		TTE	transthroacic echocardiography
NSAID	non-steroidal anti-inflammatory drug		U&E	urea and electrolytes
NSTEMI	non-ST-segment elevation myocardial infarction		VCO_2	carbon dioxide production
			VF	ventricular fibrillation
NYHA	New York Heart Association		VIE	vacuum-insulated evaporator
OCP	oral contraceptive pill		VO_2	oxygen consumption
OLV	one lung ventilation		V/Q	ventilation/perfusion ratio
OSAHS	obstructive sleep apnoea and hypopnoea syndrome		VT	ventricular tachycardia
			VTE	venous thromboembolism
OTC	over the counter		WHO	World Health Organisation
$PaCO_2$	arterial partial pressure of carbon dioxide			

Anaesthetic assessment and preparation for surgery

Tips for anaesthesia attachments

During your anaesthetic attachment, visit the anaesthetic preoperative assessment clinic and take the opportunity to:

- take a history and examine patients with particular attention to concurrent diseases that may impact on the conduct of anaesthesia;
- identify any risk factors for anaesthesia caused by any intercurrent disease processes;
- decide what further investigations are required;
- assess patients' airways and identify any potential difficulties with tracheal intubation;
- discuss an anaesthetic plan with an anaesthetist;
- witness consent being obtained for both general and regional anaesthesia;
- observe patients having echocardiography and cardiopulmonary exercise testing.

The nature of anaesthetists' training and experience makes them uniquely qualified to assess the inherent risks of anaesthetising each individual patient. Ideally, every patient should be seen by an anaesthetist prior to surgery to identify, manage, and minimize these risks. Traditionally, this occurred when the patient was admitted, usually the day before an elective surgical procedure. However, if at this time the patient was found to have any significant comorbidity, surgery was often postponed, but with insufficient time to admit a different patient, leading to wasted operating time. Increasingly, in attempts to improve efficiency, patients are admitted on the day of their planned surgical procedure. This further reduces the opportunity for an adequate anaesthetic assessment, limits the investigations that can be done and virtually prevents optimization of any comorbidities. This has led to significant changes in the preoperative management of patients undergoing elective surgery, including the introduction of clinics specifically for anaesthetic assessment. A variety of models of 'preoperative' or 'anaesthetic assessment' clinic exist; the following is intended to outline their principle functions. Those who require greater detail are advised to consult the document produced by the Association of Anaesthetists of Great Britain and Ireland (AAGBI), *Pre-operative Assessment and Patient Preparation. The Role of the Anaesthetist* (see useful information section).

Clinical Anaesthesia Lecture Notes, Fourth Edition. Carl Gwinnutt and Matthew Gwinnutt.
© 2012 John Wiley & Sons, Ltd. Published 2012 by John Wiley & Sons, Ltd.

The preoperative assessment clinic

Stage 1

Although not all patients need to be seen by an anaesthetist in a preoperative assessment clinic, all patients do need to be assessed by an appropriately trained individual. This role is frequently undertaken by nurses who may take a history, examine the patient, and order investigations (see below) according to the local protocol. The primary aim is to identify those patients at low risk of complications during anaesthesia and surgery. This includes patients who:

- have no coexisting medical problems;
- have a coexisting medical problem that is well controlled and does not impair daily activities, such as hypertension;
- do not require any, or require only baseline investigations (Table 1.1);
- have no history of, or predicted, anaesthetic difficulties;
- require surgery for which complications are minimal.

Having fulfilled these criteria, patients can then be listed for surgery. At this stage the patient will usually be given preliminary information about anaesthesia, often in the form of an explanatory leaflet. On admission patients will be seen by a member of the surgical team to ensure that there have not been any significant changes since attending the clinic, reaffirm consent and mark the surgical site if appropriate. The anaesthetist will:

- confirm the findings at the preoperative assessment;
- check the results of any baseline investigations;
- explain the options for anaesthesia appropriate for the procedure;
- obtain consent for anaesthesia;
- have the ultimate responsibility for deciding whether it is safe to proceed.

Stage 2

Clearly not all patients are as described above. Common reasons are:

- coexisting medical problems that impair activities of daily living;
- the discovery of previously undiagnosed medical problems, such as diabetes or hypertension;
- medical conditions that are less than optimally managed, such as angina, chronic obstructive pulmonary disease (COPD);
- abnormal baseline investigations.

These patients will need to be sent for further investigations – for example, an ECG, pulmonary function tests, echocardiography, or will be referred to the appropriate specialist for advice or management before being re-assessed. The findings of further investigations dictate whether or not the patient needs to be seen by an anaesthetist.

Stage 3

Patients that will need to be seen by an anaesthetist in the preoperative clinic are those who:

- have concurrent disease that impairs activities of daily living (ASA 3, see below);

Table 1.1 Baseline investigations in patients with no evidence of concurrent disease (ASA I)

Age of patient	Minor surgery	Intermediate surgery	Major surgery	Major 'plus' surgery
16–39	Nil	Nil	FBC	FBC, RFT
Consider	Nil	Nil	RFT, BS	Clotting, BS
40–59	Nil	Nil	FBC	FBC, RFT
Consider	ECG	ECG, FBC, BS	ECG, BS, RFT	ECG, BS, clotting
60–79	Nil	FBC	FBC, ECG, RFT	FBC, RFT, ECG
Consider	ECG	ECG, BS, RFT	BS, CXR	BS, clotting, CXR
≥80	ECG	FBC, ECG	FBC, ECG, RFT	FBC, RFT, ECG
Consider	FBC, RFT	RFT, BS	BS, CXR, clotting	BS, clotting, CXR

FBC: full blood count; RFT: renal function tests, to include sodium, potassium, urea and creatinine; ECG: electrocardiogram; BS: random blood glucose; CXR: chest X-ray. Clotting to include prothrombin time (PT), activated partial thromboplastin time (APTT), international normalized ratio (INR). Courtesy of National Institute for Health and Clinical Excellence.

- are known to have had previous anaesthetic difficulties, such as difficult intubation, allergies to drugs;
- are predicted to have the potential for difficulties, for example morbid obesity or a family history of prolonged apnoea after anaesthesia;
- are to undergo complex surgery with or without planned admission to the intensive care unit (ICU) postoperatively.

The consultation will allow the anaesthetist to:

- make a full assessment of the patient's medical condition;
- evaluate the results of any investigations or advice from other specialists;
- request any additional investigations;
- review any previous anaesthetics given;
- decide on the most appropriate anaesthetic technique, for example general or regional anaesthesia;
- begin the consent process, explaining and documenting:
  ○ the anaesthetic options available and the potential side-effects;
  ○ the risks associated with anaesthesia;
- discuss plans for postoperative care.

These patients will also be seen by their anaesthetist on admission, who will confirm that there have not been any significant changes since they were seen in the clinic, answer any further questions that the patient may have about anaesthesia, and obtain informed consent.

The ultimate aim of this process is to ensure that once patients are admitted for surgery, their intended procedures are not cancelled as a result of them being deemed 'unfit' or because their medical conditions have not been adequately investigated. Clearly the time between the patient being seen in the assessment clinic and the date of admission for surgery cannot be excessive; 4–6 weeks is usually acceptable.

The anaesthetic assessment

The anaesthetic assessment consists of taking a history from, and examining, each patient, followed by any appropriate investigations. When performed by non-anaesthetic staff, a protocol is often used to ensure all the relevant areas are covered. This section concentrates on features of particular relevance to the anaesthetist.

Present and past medical history

For the anaesthetist, the patient's medical history relating to the cardiovascular and respiratory systems are relatively more important.

Cardiovascular system

Enquire specifically about symptoms of:

- ischaemic heart disease;
- heart failure;
- hypertension;
- valvular heart disease;
- conduction defects, arrhythmias;
- peripheral vascular disease, previous deep venous thrombosis (DVT) or pulmonary embolus (PE).

Patients with a proven history of myocardial infarction (MI) are at a greater risk of further infarction perioperatively. The risk of reinfarction falls as the time elapsed since the original event increases. The time when the risk falls to an acceptable level, or to that of a patient with no previous history of MI, varies between patients. For a patient with an uncomplicated MI and a normal exercise tolerance test (ETT) elective surgery may only need to be delayed by 6–8 weeks. Patients should be asked about frequency, severity, and predictability of angina attacks. Frequently occurring or unpredictable attacks suggests unstable angina. This should prompt further investigation and optimization of anti-anginal therapy prior to proceeding with anaesthesia. The American Heart Association has produced guidance for perioperative cardiovascular evaluation (see useful information section).

Heart failure is one of the most important predictors of perioperative complications, mainly as an increased risk of perioperative cardiac morbidity and mortality. Its severity is best described using a recognized scale, such as the New York Heart Association classification (NYHA) (Table 1.2).

Untreated or poorly controlled hypertension may lead to exaggerated cardiovascular responses during anaesthesia. Both hypertension and hypotension can be precipitated, which increase the risk of myocardial and cerebral ischaemia.

Table 1.2 **New York Heart Association (NYHA) classification of cardiac function compared to Specific Activity Scale**

NYHA functional classification		Specific Activity Scale classification
Class I:	Cardiac disease without limitation of physical activity No fatigue, palpitations, dyspnoea or angina	Can perform activities requiring ≥7 METs Jog/walk at 5 mph, ski, play squash or basketball, shovel soil
Class II:	Cardiac disease resulting in slight limitation of physical activity Asymptomatic at rest, ordinary physical activity causes fatigue, palpitations, dyspnoea or angina	Can perform activities requiring ≥5 but <7 METs Walk at 4 mph on level ground, garden, rake, weed, have sexual intercourse without stopping
Class III:	Cardiac disease causing marked limitation of physical activity Asymptomatic at rest, less than ordinary activity causes fatigue, palpitations, dyspnoea or angina	Can perform activities requiring ≥2 but <5 METs Perform most household chores, play golf, push the lawnmower, shower
Class IV:	Cardiac disease limiting any physical activity Symptoms of heart failure or angina at rest, increased with any physical activity	Patients cannot perform activities requiring ≥2 METs Cannot dress without stopping because of symptoms; cannot perform any class III activities

The severity of hypertension will determine the action required:

- *Mild (SBP 140–159 mmHg, DBP 90–99 mmHg):* No evidence that delaying surgery for treatment affects outcome.
- *Moderate (SBP 160–179 mmHg, DBP 100–109 mmHg):* Consider review of treatment. If unchanged, requires close monitoring to avoid swings during anaesthesia and surgery.
- *Severe (SBP > 180 mmHg, DBP > 109 mmHg):* With a blood pressure this high, elective surgery should be postponed due to the significant risk of myocardial ischaemia, arrhythmias and intracerebral haemorrhage. In an emergency, it will require acute control in conjunction with invasive monitoring.

Respiratory system

Enquire specifically about symptoms of:

- COPD.
- asthma;
- infection;
- restrictive lung disease.

Patients with pre-existing lung disease are at increased risk of postoperative chest infections, particularly if they are also obese, or undergoing upper abdominal or thoracic surgery. If an acute upper respiratory tract infection is present, anaesthesia and surgery should be postponed unless it is for a life-threatening condition.

Assessment of exercise tolerance

Exercise capacity has long been recognized as a good predictor of postoperative morbidity and mortality. This is because surgery provokes similar physiological responses to exercising, namely an increase in tissue oxygen demand necessitating an increase in cardiac output and oxygen delivery. An indication of cardiac and respiratory reserves can be obtained by asking the patient about their ability to perform everyday physical activities before having to stop because of symptoms of chest pain, shortness of breath, etc. For example:

- Could you run for a bus?
- How far can you walk uphill?
- How far can you walk on the flat?
- Are you able to do the shopping?
- How many stairs can you climb before stopping?
- Are you able to do housework?
- Are you able to care for yourself?

The problem with such questions is that they are very subjective, dependent on the patient's motivation and patients often tend to overestimate their abilities!

The assessment can be made more objective by reference to The Specific Activity Scale (Table 1.2). Common physical activities are graded in terms of their metabolic equivalents of activity or 'METs', with 1 MET being the energy (or more accurately oxygen) used at rest. The more strenuous the activity, the greater the number of METs used. This is not specific for each patient but serves as a useful guide, and once again relies on the patient's assessment of their activity.

Other important considerations

- *Indigestion, heartburn and reflux:* possibility of a hiatus hernia. If exacerbated on bending forward or lying flat, this increases the risk of regurgitation and aspiration.
- *Rheumatoid disease:* limited movement of joints makes positioning for surgery difficult. Cervical spine and temporo-mandibular joint involvement may complicate airway management. There is often a chronic anaemia.
- *Diabetes:* an increased incidence of ischaemic heart disease, renal dysfunction, and autonomic and peripheral neuropathy. There is also an increased risk of perioperative complications, particularly disruption of glycaemic control, hypotension and infections.
- *Neuromuscular disorders:* poor respiratory function (forced vital capacity (FVC) < 1 L) predisposes to chest infection and increases the chance of needing ventilatory support postoperatively. Poor bulbar function predisposes to aspiration. Care is needed when using muscle relaxants. Consider regional anaesthesia.
- *Chronic renal failure:* anaemia and electrolyte abnormalities. Altered drug excretion restricts the choice of anaesthetic drugs. Surgery and dialysis treatments need to be coordinated.
- *Jaundice (associated with liver dysfunction):* coagulopathy. Altered drug metabolism and excretion. Care is needed especially with use of opioids.

Previous anaesthetics and operations

These have usually occurred in hospitals or occasionally, in the past, dental surgeries. Enquire about any perioperative problems, such as nausea, vomiting, dreams, awareness, jaundice. Ask if any information was given postoperatively, for example difficulty with intubation or delayed recovery. Whenever possible, check the records of previous anaesthetics to rule out or clarify problems such as difficulties with intubation, allergy to drugs given, or adverse reactions (such as malignant hyperpyrexia, see below). Some patients may have been issued with a 'Medic Alert' type bracelet or similar device giving details or a contact number. Details of previous surgical procedures may reveal potential anaesthetic problems, for example cardiac, pulmonary or cervical spine surgery.

Family history

All patients should be asked whether any family members have experienced problems with anaesthesia; for example, a history of prolonged apnoea suggests pseudocholinesterase deficiency (see Chapter 2), and an unexplained death suggests malignant hyperpyrexia (see Chapter 6). Elective surgery should be postponed if any conditions are identified while the patient is investigated appropriately. In the emergency situation, anaesthesia must be adjusted accordingly, for example by avoiding triggering drugs in a patient with a potential or actual family history of malignant hyperpyrexia.

Drug history and allergies

Identify all medications, both prescribed and over the counter (OTC), including complementary and alternative medicines. Patients will often forget to mention the oral contraceptive pill (OCP) and hormone replacement therapy (HRT) unless specifically asked. On the whole, the numbers of medications patients take rises with age. Many commonly prescribed drugs such as angiotensin converting enzyme inhibitors (ACE-I) can have important effects during anaesthesia. These can be identified by consulting a current British National Formulary (BNF), or the BNF website. Allergies to drugs, latex, topical preparations (e.g. iodine), adhesive dressings and foodstuffs should be noted.

Social history

- *Smoking:* ascertain the amount of tobacco smoked. This is usually calculated as the number of pack years; number of packs smoked each day multiplied by the number of years smoked. This gives an idea of the total amount smoked and allows comparison between individuals. In the long term smoking causes chronic lung disease and carcinoma but it also has a number of other important effects relevant to the perioperative period. It produces carbon monoxide, which combines with haemoglobin and reduces oxygen carriage and nicotine, which stimulates the sympathetic nervous system causing tachycardia, hypertension, and coronary artery narrowing. Cilliary function is impaired, increasing the risk of postoperative chest infections. Stopping smoking before anaesthesia reduces the risk of perioperative complications – the further in advance, the better. As a guide, stopping for eight weeks improves the airways; for two weeks reduces airway irritability and for as little as 24 hours before anaesthesia decreases carboxyhaemoglobin levels. Help and advice should be available at the preoperative assessment clinic.

- *Alcohol:* this is measured as units consumed per week; > 50 units/week causes induction of liver enzymes and tolerance to anaesthetic drugs. The risk of alcohol withdrawal syndrome postoperatively must be considered.
- *Drugs:* ask specifically about the use of drugs for recreational purposes, including type, frequency and route of administration. This group of patients is at risk of infection with hepatitis B and human immunodeficiency virus (HIV). There can be difficulty with venous access following intravenous drug abuse due to widespread thrombosis of veins. Withdrawal syndromes can occur postoperatively.
- *Pregnancy:* the date of the last menstrual period should be noted in all women of childbearing age. The anaesthetist may be the only person in theatre able to give this information if X-rays are required. Anaesthesia increases the risk of inducing a spontaneous abortion in early pregnancy. There is an increased risk of regurgitation and aspiration in late pregnancy. Elective surgery is best postponed until after delivery.

The examination

This concentrates on the cardiovascular and respiratory systems; the remaining systems are examined if problems relevant to anaesthesia have been identified in the history. At the end of the examination, the patient's airway is assessed to try and identify any potential problems. If a regional anaesthetic is planned, the appropriate anatomy (for example, lumbar spine for central neural block) is examined.

Cardiovascular system

Examine specifically for signs of:

- arrhythmias;
- heart failure;
- hypertension;
- valvular heart disease;
- peripheral vascular disease.

Don't forget to inspect the peripheral veins to identify any potential problems with IV access.

Respiratory system

Examine specifically for signs of:

- respiratory failure;
- impaired ventilation;
- collapse, consolidation, pleural effusion;
- additional or absent breath sounds.

Nervous system

Chronic disease of the peripheral and central nervous systems should be identified and any evidence of peripheral neuropathy, motor or sensory, recorded to ensure that any abnormalities postoperatively are not attributed to injury intraoperatively. It must be remembered that some disorders will affect the cardiovascular and respiratory systems, for example dystrophia myotonica and multiple sclerosis.

Musculoskeletal system

Note any restriction of movement and deformity if a patient has connective tissue disorders. Patients suffering from chronic rheumatoid disease frequently have a reduced muscle mass, peripheral neuropathies and pulmonary involvement. Particular attention should be paid to the patient's cervical spine and temporomandibular joints (see below).

The airway

The airway of all patients must be assessed, in order to try to predict those patients who may be difficult to intubate.

Observe the patient's anatomy looking specifically for:

- limitation of mouth opening;
- a receding mandible;
- position, number and health of teeth;
- size of the tongue;
- soft tissue swelling at the front of the neck;
- deviation of the larynx or trachea;
- limitations in flexion and extension of the cervical spine.

Finding any of these suggests that intubation may be more difficult. However, it must be remembered that all of these are subjective.

Some simple bedside tests can also be performed:

- *Mallampati criteria:* the patient, sitting upright, is asked to open their mouth and maximally protrude their tongue. The view of the pharyngeal structures is noted and graded I–IV (Fig. 1.1). Grades III and IV suggest difficult intubation.

- *Thyromental distance:* with the head fully extended on the neck, the distance between the bony point of the chin and the prominence of the thyroid cartilage is measured (Fig. 1.2). A distance of less than 7 cm suggests difficult intubation.
- *Calder test:* the patient is asked to protrude the mandible as far as possible. The lower incisors will either lie anterior to, aligned with, or posterior to the upper incisors. The latter two suggest reduced view at laryngoscopy.
- *Wilson score:* increasing weight, a reduction in head and neck movement, reduced mouth opening, and the presence of a receding mandible or buck-teeth all predispose to increased difficulty with intubation.

None of these tests, alone or in combination, will predict all difficult intubations. A Mallampati grade III or IV with a thyromental distance of < 7 cm will predict 80% of difficult intubations. If problems are anticipated, anaesthesia should be

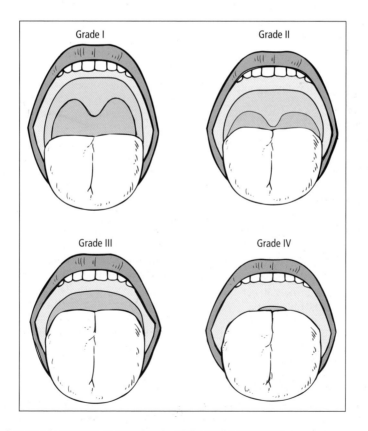

Figure 1.1 The pharyngeal structures seen during the Mallampati assessment.

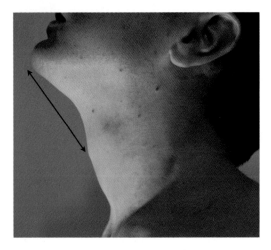

Figure 1.2   The thyromental distance.

planned accordingly. If intubation proves to be difficult, it must be recorded in a prominent place in the patient's notes and the patient informed.

Investigations

There is little evidence to support 'routine' investigations, and so an investigation should only be ordered if the result would affect the patient's management. The National Institute for Health and Clinical Excellence (NICE) produces guidelines for preoperative investigation of patients. In general, the type and number of investigations depends on the patient's age, the nature and severity of their comorbidities and the surgery planned. A synopsis of the current guidelines for *patients with no evidence of concurrent disease* (ASA 1, see below) is shown in Table 1.1. For each age group and grade of surgery, the upper entry, shows 'tests recommended' and the lower entry 'tests to be considered' (depending on patient characteristics). Dipstick urinalysis need only be performed in symptomatic individuals.

Additional investigations

The following is a guide for when to request some of the common preoperative investigations. Again the need for these will depend on the grade of surgery and the age of the patient. Further information can be found in Clinical Guideline 3, published by NICE (see useful information section).

- *Urea and electrolytes:* patients taking digoxin, diuretics, steroids, and those with diabetes, renal disease, vomiting, diarrhoea.
- *Liver function tests:* known hepatic disease, a history of a high alcohol intake (>50 units/week), metastatic disease or evidence of malnutrition.
- *Blood sugar:* diabetics, severe peripheral arterial disease or taking long-term steroids.
- *Electrocardiogram (ECG):* hypertensive, with symptoms or signs of ischaemic heart disease, a cardiac arrhythmia or diabetics > 40 years of age.
- *Chest X-ray:* symptoms or signs of cardiac or respiratory disease, or suspected or known malignancy, where thoracic surgery is planned, or in those from areas of endemic tuberculosis who have not had a chest X-ray in the last year.
- *Pulmonary function tests:* dyspnoea on mild exertion, COPD or asthma. Measure peak expiratory flow rate (PEFR), forced expiratory volume in 1 s (FEV_1) and FVC. Patients who are dyspnoeic or cyanosed at rest, found to have an $FEV_1 < 60\%$ predicted, or are to have thoracic surgery, should also have arterial blood gas analysed while breathing air.
- *Coagulation screen:* anticoagulant therapy, a history of a bleeding diatheses, or a history of liver disease or jaundice.
- *Sickle-cell screen (sickledex):* a family history of sickle-cell disease or where ethnicity increases the risk of sickle-cell disease. If positive, electrophoresis will be required for definitive diagnosis.
- *Cervical spine X-ray:* rheumatoid arthritis, a history of major trauma or surgery to the neck, or when difficult intubation is predicted.

Cardiopulmonary exercise testing

Cardiopulmonary exercise (CPX) testing objectively determines each patient's ability to increase oxygen delivery to the tissues under controlled conditions and thereby makes a preoperative assessment of their fitness. Consequently, high-risk patients can be identified allowing appropriate preparation to be made for their perioperative management.

To perform a CPX test, patients exercise using a bicycle ergometer, against an increasing resistance (like peddling uphill) while breathing through a mouthpiece. The volume and composition of inhaled and exhaled gases are monitored and analysed to determine oxygen consumption (VO_2, ml/min/kg), carbon dioxide production (VCO_2, ml/min/kg), respiratory rate, tidal volume and minute ventilation. The patient's peripheral oxygen saturation (SpO_2) and ECG are also usually monitored. The principle of the test is that, during exercise, VO_2 is the same as VCO_2. As the intensity of exercise increases, a point is reached where oxygen delivery can no longer meet metabolic demand and anaerobic metabolism starts. At this point CO_2 production exceeds oxygen consumption; this is termed the 'anaerobic threshold' (AT). If the intensity of exercise increases further, the oxygen consumption will eventually plateau (VO_2 max). This equates to the peak aerobic capacity. Many assessments of fitness measure the AT as it occurs before VO_2 max, is more easily achieved by the elderly and is less influenced by patient motivation. The lower the AT, the less cardiopulmonary reserve the patient has and the greater risk of postoperative morbidity and mortality. Table 1.3 shows values that have been used to predict risk and the need for an increased level of care postoperatively.

Unfortunately, not all patients can be assessed in this way; for example, those with severe musculoskeletal dysfunction may not be able to exercise to their anaerobic threshold. In such circumstances further investigations will be required. The most readily available method of non-invasive assessment of cardiac function in patients is some type of echocardiography (see below).

Echocardiography

This is a useful tool to assess many aspects of cardiac function in a number of diseases. In patients with heart failure or following a myocardial infarction, left ventricular function can be assessed by calculating the ejection fraction, observing the strength of contractility and looking for regional wall motion abnormalities caused by coronary artery disease. In patients with chronic pulmonary disease the right ventricular function and pulmonary artery pressures can be assessed. In patients with aortic stenosis the valve (aperture) area can be measured and the pressure gradient across the valve, which is a good indication of the severity of the disease, can be calculated. In patients with newly diagnosed atrial fibrillation, the presence of any intra-atrial blood clots can be identified. All of these things are assessed with the patient at rest and so do not give any indication of what happens when metabolic demand is increased. It is possible to simulate exercise, and hence the conditions a patient may encounter during anaesthesia or after surgery. This is often achieved by administering an inotrope, such as dobutamine, which increases heart rate and myocardial work while any changes in myocardial performance are monitored (dobutamine stress echocardiography). This is particularly useful for assessing cardiac function in patients whose exercise ability is limited, for instance by severe osteoarthritis.

Medical referral

Patients with significant medical (or surgical) comorbidities should be identified in the preoperative assessment clinic, not on the day of admission, to allow time for adequate investigation and management. Clearly a wide spectrum of conditions exists; the following are examples of some of the more commonly encountered that may need specialist advice.

Cardiovascular disease

- untreated or poorly controlled hypertension or heart failure;
- symptomatic ischaemic heart disease, despite treatment (unstable angina);
- arrhythmias: uncontrolled atrial fibrillation, paroxysmal supraventricular tachycardia, and second and third degree heart block;
- symptomatic or newly diagnosed valvular heart disease, or congenital heart disease.

Respiratory disease

- COPD, particularly if dyspnoeic at rest;
- bronchiectasis;

Table 1.3 Anaerobic threshold (AT) values used to predict risk and the need for an increased level of care postoperatively

AT >14 mL/min/kg;	no specific risk, ward based care
AT 11 – 14 mL/min/kg;	low risk, requires HDU care postoperatively
AT <11 mL/min/kg;	high risk, requires ITU care postoperatively
Basal oxygen consumption:	3.5 mL/kg/min

HDU: high dependency unit, ITU: intensive therapy unit.

- asthmatics who are unstable, taking oral steroids or have a $FEV_1 < 60\%$ predicted.

Endocrine disorders

- insulin-dependent and non-insulin-dependent diabetics who have ketonuria, glycosylated Hb (HbA1c) $> 10\%$ or a random blood sugar > 12 mmol/L. Local policy will dictate referral of stable diabetics for perioperative management;
- hypo- or hyperthyroidism symptomatic on current treatment;
- Cushing's or Addison's disease;
- hypopituitarism.

Renal disease

- chronic renal failure;
- patients undergoing renal replacement therapy.

Haematological disorders

- bleeding diatheses, for example haemophilia, thrombocytopenia;
- therapeutic anticoagulation;
- haemoglobinopathies;
- polycythaemia;
- haemolytic anaemias;
- leukaemias.

The obese patient

The degree of obesity is defined by a patient's body mass index (BMI), the ratio of weight to height and expressed in kg/m^2 (Table 1.4). An alternative definition uses waist circumference:

- overweight: > 80 cm for women, > 94 cm for men;
- obese: > 88 cm for women, > 102 cm for men.

In 2008 approximately 37% of adults in UK were overweight and 24% were obese, with a government report predicting that over 50% of adults

Table 1.4 Classification of obesity by body mass index (BMI)

Classification	BMI (kg/m²)
Healthy	20–25
Overweight	25–30
Obese	30–40
Morbidly obese	40–50 (or >35 if significant comorbidity)
Super obese	>50

will be obese by 2050 (*Tackling Obesities: The Foresight Report*). Consequently, increasing numbers of obese patients are presenting for surgery either to treat their obesity (bariatric surgery) or for unrelated surgery. Most of the principles of assessment are common to both forms of surgery. Patients with mild degrees of obesity pose few additional problems for their perioperative management. Those whose weight is greatly increased require special consideration in terms of their anatomical and physiological abnormalities and associated comorbidities when planning anaesthesia and surgery.

All patients must have their height and weight measured and their BMI calculated and recorded. Do not rely on the patient's own estimate. Specific attention should be paid to comorbidities that place obese patients at higher risk.

Cardiovascular system

Hypertension, ischaemic heart disease, hyperlipidaemia and heart failure are more common in obese patients. Although the history and examination may reveal signs and symptoms of cardiac disease, immobility often limits the patient's exercise tolerance and symptoms are not evident. A lower threshold should be used for requesting a 12-lead ECG and a stress echocardiogram may be indicated for patients who are unable to exercise sufficiently.

Respiratory system

A careful history should be taken of dyspnoea, exercise tolerance and for obstructive sleep apnoea. Pulse oximetry can easily be carried out in the preoperative clinic and a supine $SpO_2 < 96\%$ on room air suggest that further investigations (spirometry, arterial blood gases) or referral to a respiratory physician are appropriate. Morbidly obese patients with asthma or COPD are at even greater risk of perioperative respiratory complications. Wheeze in obese patients may be due to airway closure rather than asthma. Pulmonary function tests before and after bronchodilator therapy may be useful in differentiation between the two conditions. Obstructive sleep apnoea and hypopnoea syndrome (OSAHS) are common in this group of patients. Those who have symptoms of daytime sleepiness should complete an Epworth sleepiness assessment (Table 1.5). If positive (score > 10), they should be referred for further

Table 1.5 Epworth sleepiness assessment. Each category is scored: 0 = would never doze or sleep, 1 = slight chance of dozing or sleeping, 2 = moderate chance of dozing or sleeping, 3 = high chance of dozing or sleeping. The total of the scores is summed, >10 is considered abnormal

- Sitting and reading
- Watching TV
- Sitting inactive in a public place
- As a passenger in a car for an hour without a break
- Lying down in the afternoon when circumstances permit
- Sitting and talking to someone
- Sitting quietly after lunch without alcohol
- In a car stopped for a few minutes in traffic

investigations and consideration of continuous positive airway pressure (CPAP) or bi-level positive airway pressure (BiPAP) therapy preoperatively. Intubation may be more difficult because of deposition of fat into the soft tissues of the neck – a full assessment of the airway is mandatory.

Metabolic and gastrointestinal systems

Morbidly obese patients have a high incidence of diabetes mellitus. All patients should be questioned about symptoms of diabetes and have appropriate investigations if symptomatic. Those known to be diabetic should be assessed for the adequacy of glucose control, for example HbA1c, and also for the presence of complications, especially coronary artery disease, diabetic nephropathy and autonomic dysfunction. Improved perioperative glucose control may help reduce complications such as wound infections or the development of keto- or lactic acidosis. Ask about symptoms of acid reflux, appropriate antacid prophylaxis may be indicated preoperatively.

Other issues

Preoperative assessment several weeks prior to planned surgery will allow the opportunity to optimize the patient's medical comorbidities, plan for anaesthesia, and arrange the appropriate level of postoperative care. All of these may be more complicated than for patients of normal weight. Informed consent should be obtained with discussion of any specific increased risks

related to anaesthesia. Following full assessment and an explanation of the potential risks, some patients may reconsider whether or not to proceed with surgery.

Risk associated with anaesthesia and surgery

One of the most commonly asked questions of anaesthetists is *'What are the risks of having an anaesthetic?'* The Royal College of Anaesthetists and the AAGBI have issued a guide for patients titled *You and Your Anaesthetic*. This divides the risks associated with anaesthesia and their frequency:

Common (1 in 10 to 1 in 100)

These are not life threatening and can occur even when anaesthesia has apparently been uneventful. They include:

- bruising and soreness from attempts at IV access;
- sore throat;
- headache;
- dizziness;
- postoperative nausea and vomiting;
- itching;
- retention of urine.

Uncommon (1 in 1000)

- dental damage;
- chest infection;
- muscle pains;
- an existing condition worsening, such as myocardial infarction;
- awareness during general anaesthesia.

Rare (<1 in 10000)

- allergy to the anaesthetic drugs;
- eye injury, particularly if prone;
- nerve damage;
- hypoxic brain injury;
- death.

In the United Kingdom, the Confidential Enquiry into Perioperative Deaths (CEPOD 1987) revealed an *overall* perioperative mortality of 0.7% in approximately 500 000 operations. Anaesthesia was considered to have been a contributing factor in 410 deaths (0.08%), but was judged *completely* responsible in only three cases–a primary mortality rate of 1:185 000 operations. Upon analysis of the deaths where anaesthesia contributed, the predominant factor was human error.

Clearly, anaesthesia itself is very safe, particularly in those patients who are otherwise well. Apart from human error, the most likely major risk is from an adverse drug reaction or drug interaction. However, anaesthesia rarely occurs in isolation and when the risks of the surgical procedure and those due to pre-existing disease are combined, the risks of morbidity and mortality are increased. Not surprisingly a number of methods have been described to try to quantify these risks.

Risk indicators

The most widely used scale for estimating risk is the ASA classification of the patient's physical status. The patient is assigned to a category from one to five depending on any physical disturbance caused by either the disease process for which surgery is being performed, or any other pre-existing disease. It is relatively subjective, which leads to a degree of variability between scorers. Different studies have reported different mortalities for each grade. This is a result of differences in; populations of patients, sample sizes, types of

surgery being performed and the duration of monitoring patients postoperatively, for example deaths at 48 hours or at one week. However, patients placed in higher categories are at increased overall risk of perioperative mortality (Table 1.6).

The leading cause of death after surgery is myocardial infarction, and significant morbidity results from non-fatal infarction, particularly in patients with pre-existing heart disease. As well as the risks from pre-existing cardiac disease, different operations also carry their own varying levels of inherent risks; for example carpal tunnel decompression carries less risk than a hip replacement, which in turn carries less risk than aortic aneurysm surgery. Basically this can be summarized as 'the sicker the patient and the bigger the operation, the greater the risk.'

Assessing patients as 'low risk' is no more of a guarantee that complications will not occur than 'high risk' means they will occur; it is only a guideline and indicator of probability. For patients who suffer a complication the rate is 100%! Ultimately the risk/benefit ratio must be considered for each individual patient. If a patient has a certain predicted risk of complications, an operation with the potential to offer only a small benefit may be deemed not worth the risk, whereas one with the potential to offer a large benefit may in fact be undertaken. Clearly this is a decision that can only be reached after careful

Table 1.6 **ASA physical status scale**		
Class	**Physical status**	**Absolute mortality (%)**
I	A healthy patient with no organic or psychological disease process. The pathological process for which the operation is being performed is localized and causes no systemic upset	0–0.3
II	A patient with a mild to moderate systemic disease process, caused by the condition to be treated surgically or another pathological process, that does not limit the patient's activities in any way e.g. treated hypertensive, stable diabetic. Patients aged >80 years are automatically placed in class II	0.3–1.4
III	A patient with severe systemic disease from any cause that imposes a definite functional limitation on activity e.g. ischaemic heart disease, COPD	1.5–5.4
IV	A patient with a severe systemic disease that is a constant threat to life, e.g. unstable angina	7.8–25.9
V	A moribund patient unlikely to survive 24 hours with or without surgery	9.4–57.8
VI	A patient declared brain dead whose organs are being removed for transplantation	

Note: 'E' may be added to signify an emergency operation.

and thorough discussion with a patient who has been given all the relevant information.

Improving preoperative preparation by optimizing the patient's physical status, adequately resuscitating those who require emergency surgery, appropriate intraoperative monitoring, and by providing suitable postoperative care in an appropriate level of critical care, has been shown to further reduce patients perioperative mortality.

Classification of operation

Traditionally, surgery was classified as being either elective or emergency. Recognizing that this was too imprecise, the National Confidential Enquiry into Perioperative Outcome and Death (NCEPOD) has identified four categories:

1 Immediate: to save life, limb or organ. Resuscitation is simultaneous with surgery. The target time to theatre is within minutes of the decision that surgery is necessary – for example, major trauma to the abdomen or thorax with uncontrolled haemorrhage, major neurovascular deficit, ruptured aortic aneurysm.
2 Urgent: acute onset or deterioration of a condition that threatens life, limb or organ. Surgery normally takes place when resuscitation is complete. Examples would be compound fracture, perforated viscus, cauda equina syndrome. This category is subdivided into:
   2A. Target time to theatre within 6 hours of the decision to operate
   2B. Target time to theatre within 24 hours of the decision to operate
3 Expedited: stable patient requiring early intervention. Condition not an immediate threat to life, limb or organ. Target time to theatre is within days of the decision to operate. Examples would be closed fracture, tendon injury, some tumour surgery.
4 Elective: surgery planned and booked in advance of admission to hospital. This category includes all conditions not covered in categories 1–3. Typical examples would be joint replacements, cholecystectomy, hernia repair.

All elective and the majority of expedited cases can be assessed as previously described. In urgent and emergency cases this will not always be possible, but as much information as possible should be obtained about allergies, the patient's medical history, drugs taken regularly and previous anaesthetics. In the trauma patient, enquire about the mechanism of injury. This may give clues to unsuspected injuries. Details may only be available from relatives and/or the ambulance crew. The cardiovascular and respiratory systems should be examined and an assessment made of any potential difficulty with intubation. Investigations should only be ordered if they would directly affect the conduct of anaesthesia. When life or limb is at stake, there will be even less or no time for assessment. All emergency patients should be assumed to have a full stomach.

Prevention of venous thromboembolism

Up to 25 000 patients die each year in the UK as a result of a hospital-acquired venous thromboembolism (VTE). It is now a requirement that all patients admitted to hospital are assessed for their risk of developing a VTE and appropriate preventative measures applied. Surgical patients and patients with trauma are at increased risk of VTE with:

- a total anaesthetic and surgical time > 90 min;
- surgery to the pelvis or lower limb and the total anaesthetic and surgical time > 60 min;
- an acute surgical admission with inflammatory or intra-abdominal condition;
- an expected reduction in mobility.

Further non-surgical factors increase the risk of VTE:

- active cancer or treatment for cancer;
- age > 60 years;
- critical care admission;
- dehydration;
- known thrombophilia;
- BMI > 30 $kg\,m^{-2}$;
- one or more significant medical comorbidities (for example, heart disease, respiratory disease, endocrine or metabolic disorders);
- personal or first-degree relative with a history of VTE;
- use of HRT;
- use of oestrogen containing contraceptive;
- varicose veins with phlebitis.

Patients must also be assessed for their risk of bleeding:

- active bleeding;
- acquired coagulopathy (for example, liver failure);

- concurrent anticoagulation;
- epidural, spinal anaesthesia (or lumbar puncture) within the last 4 hours or expected within 12 hours;
- acute stroke;
- thrombocytopaenia;
- uncontrolled hypertension (>230/120 mmHg);
- untreated bleeding disorders (for example, haemophilia).

Where the risks of VTE exceed the risks of bleeding, VTE prophylaxis should be used. The method used will depend upon the type and site of surgery and may be mechanical (for example, anti-embolism stockings, pneumatic calf compression) or pharmacological (for example, heparin, fondiparinux, or rivaroxaban). All patients should be reassessed 24 h after admission to identify any clinical changes, to ensure that the method chosen has been implemented and to identify any adverse effects.

Obtaining informed consent

What is consent?

It is an agreement by the patient to undergo a specific procedure. Even though the doctor will advise on what is required, it is only the patient who can make the decision to undergo the procedure. Although the need for consent is often thought of as applying to surgery, it is in fact required for any breach of a patient's personal integrity, including examination, performing investigations, and giving an anaesthetic. Touching a patient without consent may lead to a claim of battery. Consent may be explicit or expressed, for example when a person agrees, either verbally or in writing. Consent can also be implied as indicated by an informed patient's behaviour, but this form of consent only has validity if the patient genuinely knows and understands what is being proposed. An example would be a patient voluntarily holding an arm out for a blood test after an explanation of why the test is needed. Whatever form of consent is obtained, providing sufficient, accurate information is essential. When patients do not know what is proposed, or are unaware that they can refuse, they have not given consent. In medicine, when obtaining

consent for an operation or invasive procedure it is written, explicit consent that is most commonly used.

All people aged 16 years and over are presumed, in law, to have the capacity to consent to treatment unless there is evidence to the contrary. Suffering from a mental disorder or impairment does not automatically mean lack of competence. Some patients who would normally be considered competent may be temporarily incapable of giving valid consent due to intoxication from drugs or alcohol, severe pain or shock. A decision that appears to be irrational or unjustified should not be taken as evidence that the individual lacks the mental capacity to make that decision.

For a patient to have the capacity to give valid consent there are five prerequisites. They should:

- understand what is being proposed, its purpose and why it is being proposed;
- understand the benefits, risks and any alternatives;
- understand the consequences of not receiving what is being proposed;
- retain the information long enough to arrive at a decision;
- be able to communicate their decision.

The decision the patient makes does not have to appear sensible or rational to anybody else. However, every effort must be made to ensure that a highly irrational decision is not the result of a lack of, or misinterpretation of, the information given. It may of course also indicate that the patient is suffering from a mental illness. Determining capacity in these circumstances is probably best placed in the hands of the courts.

Refusal of treatment by a competent adult is legally binding (except where the law states otherwise, for example under mental health legislation), even if refusal is likely to lead to the patient's death (for example, a Jehovah's Witness refusing a blood transfusion). Although a patient can refuse treatment or choose a less-than-optimal option, they cannot insist on a treatment that has not been offered.

What do I have to tell the patient?

Although the anaesthetist is the best judge of the type of anaesthetic for each individual, where there is a choice patients should be given an explanation along with the associated risks and benefits of the options. The amount of information given to patients can often be determined by asking oneself 'what would *this* patient regard as relevant when coming to a decision about which, if any, of the available options to accept?' A balance is required between listening to what the patient wants and providing enough information, in terms that the patient can understand, in order that the patient's decisions are informed.

Typical information regarding anaesthesia may be:

- the environment of the anaesthetic room and who patients will meet, particularly if medical students or other healthcare professionals in training will be present;
- the need for intravenous access and IV infusion (a drip);
- the need for, and type of, any invasive monitoring;
- what to expect during a regional technique;
- being conscious throughout surgery if a regional technique alone is used and what they may hear;
- preoxygenation;
- use of cricoid pressure;
- induction of anaesthesia; although most commonly intravenous, occasionally it may be by inhalation;
- where they will 'wake up' – this is usually the recovery unit, but after some surgery it may be in a critical care area (in these circumstances the patient should be given the opportunity to visit the unit a few days before and meet some of the staff);
- numbness and loss of movement after regional anaesthesia;
- the possibility of drains, catheters and drips – patients may misinterpret their presence as indicating unexpected problems;
- the possibility of a need for blood transfusion;
- postoperative pain control, particularly if it requires their co-operation – for example, a patient-controlled analgesia device (see Chapter 7);
- information on any substantial risks associated with the anaesthetic technique (see above).

Most patients will want to know the latest time that they can eat and drink before surgery, if they should take their medications as normal, and how they will manage without a drink. The Royal College of Anaesthetists and AAGBI recommend that in patients with normal gastric emptying, the evidence is that clear fluids empty rapidly and consequently day cases and inpatients can be allowed clear fluids for up to 2 hours before anaesthesia. This will not include patients with conditions that delay gastric emptying, for example, trauma, pain, or gastrointestinal disease, and where there is use of opioid drugs. The evidence for solids is less clear but consensus opinion is a period of 6 hours fasting after a light meal, milk, or drinks containing milk is acceptable. Some will expect or request a premed and in these circumstances the approximate timing, route of administration, and likely effects should be discussed. Finally, before leaving, ask if the patient has any questions or wants anything clarifying further.

Having given the patient the information considered relevant to them, they must have sufficient time to think it through and come to a decision. Consequently, the process of informed consent cannot occur solely at the point of admission, or even worse, in the anaesthetic room immediately before surgery! As a result, the process usually starts in the preoperative assessment clinic when information is often given to the patient in the form of a leaflet, such as *You and Your Anaesthetic*, published jointly by the Royal College of Anaesthetists and the AAGBI.

Who should get consent?

From the above it is clear that the individual seeking consent must be able to provide all the necessary information for the patient and be able to answer the patient's questions. This will require the individual to be trained in, and familiar with, the procedure for which consent is sought, and is best done by a senior clinician or the person who is to perform the procedure. Complex problems may require a multidisciplinary approach to obtaining consent.

Where there has been a significant interval between obtaining consent for the procedure and start of treatment, or if new information is available, consent should be reaffirmed. The aim is to provide any new information and allow patients the opportunity to ask questions and to review their decision. This process may be delegated to a doctor who is trained, qualified and familiar with the procedure, who can answer the patient's questions.

The issues around consent in children and adults who lack capacity are more complex. Further information is available in the document *Consent for Anaesthesia*, published by the AAGBI (see useful information section).

What constitutes evidence of consent?

Most patients will be asked to sign a consent form before undergoing a procedure. However, there is no legal requirement for this before anaesthesia or surgery (or anything else). Consent may be given verbally and this is often the case for anaesthesia, however it is recommended that a written record of the content of the conversation be made in the patient's case notes.

What about an unconscious patient?

This usually arises in the emergency situation, for example a patient with a severe head injury. Asking a relative or other individual to sign a consent form for surgery on the patient's behalf is not appropriate, as no one can give consent on behalf of another adult. Under these circumstances, if an intervention is required to save a patient's life or avoid significant deterioration in their health before they will regain capacity to consent, medical staff are required to act 'in the patient's best interests'. This will mean taking into account not only the benefits of the proposed treatment but also personal and social factors. Such information may necessitate a discussion with relatives, and the opportunity should be used to inform them of the proposed treatment and the rationale for it. Where there is clear evidence of a valid advance refusal by an adult of a particular treatment (such as a refusal of blood by a Jehovah's Witness) then that treatment must not be given. If a patient has appointed a welfare attorney, or there is a court-appointed deputy or guardian, where practicable this individual must be consulted about any proposed treatment.

The basis for any decision and how it is in the patient's best interests must be clearly documented in the patient's notes. Where treatment decisions are complex or not clear cut, it is advisable although not a legal requirement, to obtain and document independent medical advice.

For more detail on consent, the reader is strongly encouraged to refer to the *Consent Tool Kit*, 5th edn, published by the British Medical Association and available on their website (see useful information section).

📖 FURTHER USEFUL INFORMATION

Wolters U, Wolf T, Stutzer H and Schroder T. ASA classification and perioperative variables as predictors of postoperative outcome. *British Journal of Anaesthesia* 1996; **77**: 217–222.

www.aagbi.org/publications/guidelines/docs/consent06.pdf
[Consent for anesthesia. Revised edition 2006. The Association of Anaesthetists of Great Britain and Ireland.]

www.aagbi.org/publications/guidelines/docs/preop2010.pdf
[Pre-operative assessment and patient preparation. The role of the anaesthetist. The Association of Anaesthetists of Great Britain and Ireland. November 2010.]

www.bma.org.uk/ethics/consent_and_capacity/consenttoolkit.jsp
[BMA consent toolkit, 5th edn, December 2009.]

www.BNF.org
[British National Formulary.]

http://www.circ.ahajournals.org/cgi/content/full/116/17/1971
[American College of Cardiology/American Heart Association (ACC/AHA) Guideline Update on Perioperative Cardiovascular Evaluation for Noncardiac Surgery. 2002.]

http://circ.ahajournals.org/content/120/21/2123.full.pdf
[ACC/AHA 2006 Guideline Update on Perioperative Cardiovascular Evaluation for Noncardiac Surgery: Focused Update on Perioperative Beta-Blocker Therapy. A Report of the American College of Cardiology/American Heart Association Task Force on Practice Guidelines (Writing Committee to Update the 2002 Guidelines on Perioperative Cardiovascular Evaluation for Noncardiac Surgery).]

http://www.dh.gov.uk/en/Publicationsandstatistics/Publications/PublicationsPolicyAndGuidance/DH_103643
[Department of Health (UK) guidance on consent.]

http://www.legislation.gov.uk/ukpga/2005/9/
contents
[Mental capacity Act 2005. Department of
Constitutional Affairs.]
www.ncepod.org.uk/
[The National Confidential Enquiry into Patient
Outcome and Death (NCEPOD).]
http://guidance.nice.org.uk/CG3/NICEGuidance/
pdf/English
[National Institute for Health and Clinical

Excellence (NICE) guidance on preoperative
tests. June 2003.]
www.pre-op.org/index.html
[The Preoperative Association.]
www.youranaesthetic.info/
[Patient information guides from the Association of Anaesthetists of Great Britain and Ireland and The Royal College of Anaesthetists.]

All websites last accessed February 2012.

? SELF-ASSESSMENT

Short-answer questions

1.1 Describe three methods of assessing a patient's exercise capacity preoperatively.

1.2 Describe the bedside assessments that you could use to try and predict difficulty with tracheal intubation.

1.3 Describe the characteristics that define each of the ASA grades. What ASA grade would you assign to a 67-year-old woman with type II diabetes, hypertension, a BMI of 38 and exercise tolerance of 100 m on the flat and why?

1.4 In the preoperative assessment clinic, what investigations would you do on a 70-year-old woman, with controlled hypertension and COPD from smoking 20 cigarettes per day for 50 years, who is scheduled for a total hip replacement and why?

1.5 A 43-year-old woman seen in the clinic prior to having a laparoscopic cholecystectomy is assessed as being ASA II due to well controlled hypertension. She asks 'what are the risks of having a general anaesthetic?' What would you tell her?

True/false questions

1.1 A 49-year-old woman is seen in the preop clinic, prior to having a laparoscopic cholecystectomy. She has a $BMI = 39\,kg/m^2$, type 2 diabetes and hypertension. She is currently taking metformin, ramipril, aspirin and simvastatin. She will require the following investigations:
 a 12-lead ECG;
 b chest X-ray;
 c FBC, U + Es;
 d coagulation screen.

1.2 Difficulty with tracheal intubation is suggested by finding:
 a A thyromental distance of > 7 cm;
 b With the patient's mouth fully open, inability to see the posterior wall of the pharynx;
 c Ability by the patient to protrude the lower incisors beyond the upper incisors;
 d A BMI of > 35 kg/m^2.

1.3 The following are common risks (1:10 to 1:100) of anaesthesia:
 a postoperative nausea and vomiting;
 b urinary retention;
 c dental damage;
 d allergy to the anaesthetic drugs.

1.4 The following factors increase the risk of VTE:
 a age > 50 years;
 b BMI > 30 kg/m^2;
 c taking HRT;
 d lower limb surgery lasting > 60 min.

1.5 In the assessment of the cardiovascular system:
 a a patient with a preoperative blood pressure of 184/116 mmHg should have elective surgery delayed until the blood pressure is under control;
 b echocardiography can quantify the severity of heart valve dysfunction;
 c echocardiography can be used to assess ventricular function during pharmacologically simulated exercise;
 d cardiopulmonary exercise (CPX) testing assesses the patient's ability to increase carbon dioxide clearance during exercise.

2

Anaesthetic equipment and monitoring

Anaesthesia is a very practical specialty and, to practise safely, anaesthetists must be familiar with the equipment used. This ranges from the simple to the technical and its complexity is increasing relentlessly. The following is an overview of the equipment and monitoring currently in use. No excuse is made for including very simple devices; these are often the most valuable but if used wrongly may endanger the patient's safety.

Airway equipment

The ability to ensure that a patient has a patent airway at all times is arguably the most important skill that an anaesthetist possesses. There is an ever increasing range of airway conduits and equipment to aid their insertion available to the anaesthetist. The safe and efficient use of the various devices relies on some common knowledge, for example of airway anatomy, but also skills unique to the equipment being used. It would be impossible to cover in detail all the currently available airway equipment, and unrealistic to expect someone to be skilled in the use of every device available. The important thing is to know when and how to use a selected range of devices well. The following is a description of most of the commonly available airway equipment; a description of the skills needed to use it safely and successfully is given in Chapter 4.

Facemasks

These are designed to fit closely to the contours of the face and a gas-tight fit is achieved by an air-filled cuff around the edge. Traditionally these devices were made from black rubber and were reusable – the BOC anatomical facemask is an example – and required disinfection between each patient. Increasingly they are now single use and are made from transparent plastics, allowing visualization of vomit, making them popular for use during resuscitation (Fig. 2.1).

Clinical Anaesthesia Lecture Notes, Fourth Edition. Carl Gwinnutt and Matthew Gwinnutt.
© 2012 John Wiley & Sons, Ltd. Published 2012 by John Wiley & Sons, Ltd.

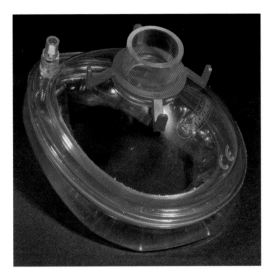

Figure 2.1 Plastic, disposable facemask.

Simple adjuncts

The oropharyngeal (Guedel) airway, and to a lesser extent the nasopharyngeal airway, are often used to help maintain the airway immediately after the induction of anaesthesia. However, their use does not guarantee a patent airway.

Oropharyngeal airway

These are curved plastic tubes, flattened in cross-section and flanged at the oral end (Fig. 2.2). They lie over the tongue, and prevent it from falling back into the pharynx. They are manufactured in a variety of sizes and suitable for all patients, from neonates to large adults. The commonest sizes are 2–4, for small to large adults, respectively. The size required is estimated by comparing the airway length with the vertical distance

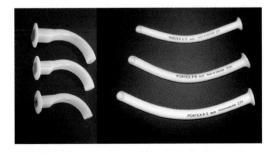

Figure 2.2 Oropharyngeal and nasopharyngeal airways.

between the patient's incisor teeth and the angle of the jaw.

Nasopharyngeal airway

These are round, malleable plastic tubes, bevelled at the pharyngeal end and flanged at the nasal end (Fig. 2.2). They lie along the floor of the nose and curve round into the pharynx. They are sized according to their internal diameter in millimetres, and their length increases with the diameter. They are not commonly used in children, and sizes 6–8 mm in diameter are suitable for small to large adults, respectively. The correct size is estimated by made by comparing the airway diameter with that of the external nares.

Supraglottic devices

In recent years there has been an increase in the number of different types of these airway devices available. They are all variations on a similar theme with various modifications to try and improve their suitability for wider applications.

The laryngeal mask airway (LMA)

This was the original supraglottic airway device and, as its name suggests, it consists of a 'mask' that sits over the laryngeal opening. This is attached to a tube that protrudes from the mouth and connects directly to the anaesthetic breathing system. Around the perimeter of the mask is an inflatable cuff that helps to stabilize it and creates a seal around the laryngeal inlet. The LMA is suitable for use in all patients, from neonates to adults, as it is produced in a variety of sizes. The most commonly used in female and male adults are sizes 3, 4 and 5. They were originally designed for use in spontaneously breathing patients but it is possible to ventilate patients via the LMA. When doing this care must be taken to avoid high inflation pressures, otherwise leakage occurs past the cuff, reducing ventilation and potentially causing gastric inflation. The original LMA (or classic LMA) is a reusable device requiring sterilization between each patient, but recent concerns about the possible risk of prion disease transmission have resulted in increasing use of disposable versions (Fig. 2.3a).

There have been a number of modifications to the LMA:

- A version with a more flexible and reinforced tube. This is useful in maxillo-facial or ear, nose

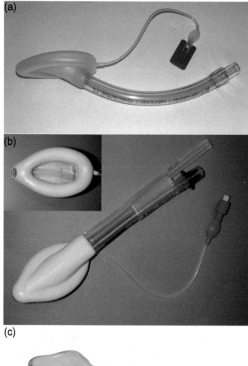

(a)

(b)

(c)

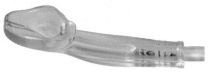

Figure 2.3 Supraglottic airway devices. (a) Disposable LMA, (b) LMA Pro-Seal™, (c) i-gel™.

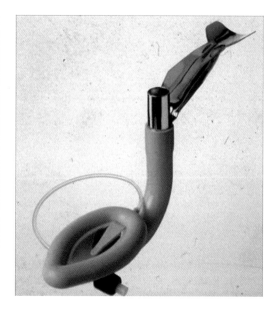

Figure 2.4 Intubating Laryngeal Mask Airway (ILMA®).

and throat surgery as it allows the tube part to be flexed and directed out of the surgeon's way without kinking and occlusion of the lumen.

- The LMA Pro-Seal™ (Fig. 2.3b). This has an additional posterior cuff to improve the seal between mask and larynx, and reduce leak when the patient is ventilated. It also has a secondary tube to allow drainage of gastric contents.
- The i-gel™ (Fig. 2.3c). This is the latest development which uses a solid, highly malleable, gel-like material contoured to fit the perilaryngeal anatomy in place of the traditional inflatable cuff. It is single use.
- The intubating LMA (Fig. 2.4). As the name suggests, this device is used as a conduit to perform tracheal intubation without the need for laryngoscopy (see below).

The intubating LMA (ILMA)

This is a modification of the LMA in which the mask part is almost unchanged, but a shorter, wider metal tube with a 90° bend in it with a handle replaces the flexible tube (Fig. 2.4). It is inserted using a similar technique as for a standard LMA, but by holding the handle rather than using one's index finger as a guide. A specially designed reinforced, cuffed, tracheal tube can then be inserted, which will almost always pass into the trachea, due to the shape and position of the ILMA. Once it has been confirmed that the tube lies in the trachea, the ILMA can either be left in place or removed. This device has proved to be very popular in cases where direct laryngoscopy does not give a good view of the larynx and tracheal intubation fails. The most recent development is the C-Trach®, in which the larynx is viewed from the mask aperture using/via a fibre optic cable attached to a small monitor positioned at the proximal end of the device (Fig. 2.5).

Tracheal tubes

These are manufactured from plastic (PVC), are single use to eliminate cross-infection, and are sized according to their internal diameter. They are available in a range of sizes at 0.5 mm diameter intervals making them suitable for use in all patients from neonates to adults, and are long

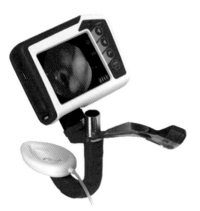

Figure 2.5 C-Trach®: an ILM with integrated fibre optics to allow an indirect view of the larynx.

enough to be used orally or nasally. A standard 15 mm connector is provided to allow connection to the breathing system.

The tracheal tubes used during adult anaesthesia have an inflatable cuff to prevent leakage of anaesthetic gases back past the tube when positive pressure ventilation is used, and also to prevent aspiration of any foreign material into the lungs. The cuff is inflated by injecting air via a pilot tube, at the distal end of which is a one-way valve to prevent deflation and a small 'balloon' to indicate when the cuff is inflated. A wide variety of specialized tubes have been developed, examples of which are shown in Fig. 2.6a–d.

- *Reinforced tubes:* used to prevent kinking and subsequent obstruction as a result of the positioning of the patient's head.
- *Preformed tubes:* used during surgery on the head and neck, and are designed to take the connections away from the surgical field.
- *Double lumen tubes:* effectively two tubes welded together side-by-side, with one tube extending distally beyond the other. They are used during thoracic surgery, and allow one

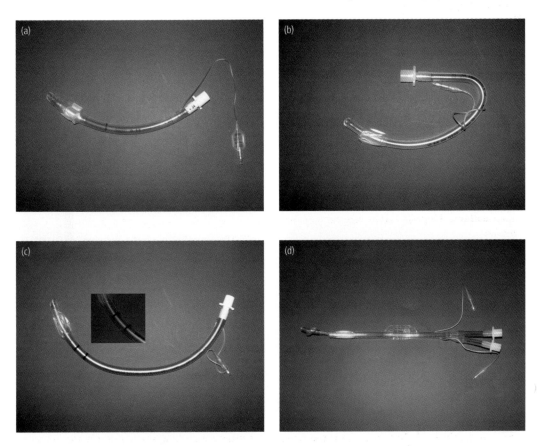

Figure 2.6 Tracheal tubes: (a) standard, (b) preformed (RAE tube), (c) reinforced tube, (d) double lumen tube.

lung to be deflated whilst ventilation is maintained via the bronchial portion in the opposite lung.

• *Uncuffed tubes:* used in children up to approximately 8 years of age as the narrowing in the subglottic region provides a natural seal. (Specialized cuffed tubes for children below this age are used in some paediatric units.)

Laryngoscopes

Direct

These are the traditional laryngoscopes, designed to allow direct visualization of the larynx to facilitate the insertion of a tracheal tube. They consist of a blade with a light at the tip, attached to a handle that contains the batteries for the light. The most popular type in use is the curved blade designed by, and named after, Sir Robert Macintosh (Fig. 2.7a). Different sized blades are available. There have been many developments in the design of this device, and one of the most successful is the McCoy blade (Figs 2.7b and c). This has a flexible tip operated by a lever adjacent to the handle that increases the elevation of the epiglottis to improve the view of the larynx. Occasionally a straight-bladed laryngoscope may be used, such as the Magill blade.

Indirect

Recently, numerous devices have been developed that make use of advanced optics and electronics in order to overcome the difficulties when the larynx cannot be directly visualized using the

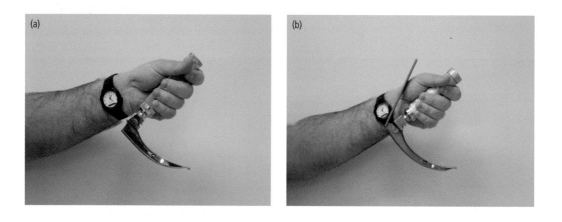

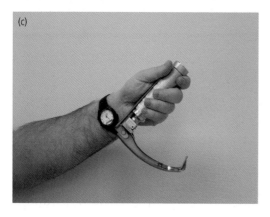

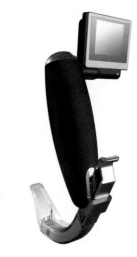

Figure 2.7 Laryngoscopes: (a) Macintosh, (b) McCoy, (c) McCoy with tip flexed, (d) McGrath.

laryngoscopes described above. The operator can visualize the larynx either by 'looking through' these devices or by having the image displayed on a separate screen. Some examples that highlight the different technologies used are included here:

- Videolaryngoscopes, for example the McGrath Scope (Fig. 2.7d). There are several of these devices available from different manufacturers. They are more like a conventional laryngoscope except that they have a small camera at the tip. This image is displayed on a small screen and allows a better view of the larynx. Also, some of them have modified shaped blades or tracheal tube guides to help with tube placement. These devices may also have a role to play in training as a supervisor can see what the student sees and offer advice and guidance to improve technique.
- Fibreoptic bronchoscope (Fig. 2.8). A narrow diameter flexible bronchoscope that transmits the image from the tip of the scope via thousands of small diameter glass fibres to an eye piece or a display monitor. The tip is manoeuvrable from the handle to help guide the scope in the right direction, and there is a suction channel to remove any secretions from the airways. An appropriate size and length tracheal tube is loaded onto the bronchoscope which is then inserted into either the nose or the mouth and advanced until it lies in the trachea. Once the tip of the bronchoscope is inside the trachea the tracheal tube is passed over the scope until it is seen to pass the tip of the scope and also lie in the trachea. Then the bronchoscope is removed and the tracheal tube cuff is inflated and it is connected to the breathing system. This procedure can be done with the patient

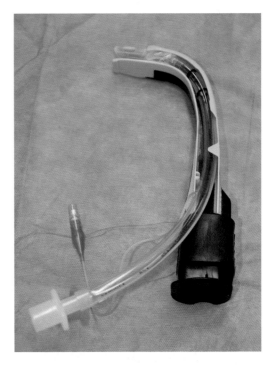

Figure 2.9 Airtraq®, a single-use device for intubation. Allows an indirect view of the larynx and has a guide to insert the tracheal tube.

awake, following suitable sedation and airway anaesthesia, or with the patient anaesthetised.

- Airtraq® (Fig. 2.9). This device uses a prism to aid with visualizing the larynx, and a slot on the side into which the tracheal tube is inserted that helps with placement of the tube.
- Optical stylets (Fig. 2.10). Very similar in principle to the flexible fibre optic bronchoscope except that they are rigid, and only suitable for oral use in patients under general anaesthesia.

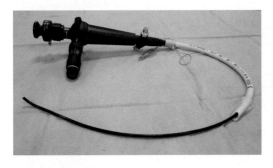

Figure 2.8 Fibreoptic intubating bronchoscope. A tracheal tube has been mounted ready to advance into the trachea.

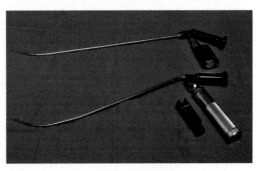

Figure 2.10 Optical stylets. Bonfils (above), Shikani (below).

Gum elastic bougie

This is a 60 cm-long malleable introducer, with a slightly angled tip. Its construction allows it to be bent into a gentle curve before it is introduced so that it can be directed blindly behind the epiglottis into the trachea. It is then rigid enough to allow a tracheal tube to be passed over it.

The safe delivery of anaesthesia

The delivery of gases to the operating theatre

Most hospitals use a piped medical gas and vacuum system (PMGV) to distribute oxygen, nitrous oxide, medical air and vacuum. The pipelines' outlets act as self-closing sockets, each specifically configured, coloured and labelled for one gas. Oxygen, nitrous oxide and air are delivered to the anaesthetic room at a pressure of 400 kilopascals (kPa) (4 bar, 60 pounds per square inch (psi)). The gases (and vacuum) reach the anaesthetic machine via flexible reinforced hoses, colour-coded throughout their length (oxygen – white, nitrous oxide – blue, vacuum – yellow). These attach to the wall outlet via a gas-specific probe and to the anaesthetic machine via a gas-specific nut and union. Cylinders are used as reserves in case of pipeline failure. The gas content has traditionally been indicated by the colour of the body and shoulder of the cylinder (Table 2.1), although the contents must always be confirmed by checking the attached label. However, recent legislation has proposed that all medical gas cylinders should have a white body with coloured shoulders (Table 2.1). This

change will occur gradually, being complete by 2025. In the interim period, to limit errors, the content will be written on the body of all cylinders. All cylinders have a pin-index safety mechanism to prevent the connection of the wrong cylinder to the wrong terminal on the anaesthetic machine.

Oxygen

Piped oxygen is supplied from a liquid oxygen reserve, where it is stored under pressure (7–10 bar, 1000 kPa) at approximately minus 160 °C in a vacuum-insulated evaporator (VIE), effectively a large thermos flask. Gaseous oxygen is removed from above the liquid, or at times of increased demand, by vaporizing liquid oxygen using heat from the environment. The gas is warmed to ambient air temperature en route from the VIE to the pipeline system. A reserve bank of cylinders of compressed oxygen is kept adjacent to the VIE in case the main system fails. A smaller cylinder is attached directly to the anaesthetic machine as an emergency reserve. The pressure in a full cylinder is of oxygen is 13 700 kPa (137 bar, 2000 psi) and this falls proportionally as the cylinder empties.

Nitrous oxide

Piped nitrous oxide is supplied from several large cylinders joined together to form a bank and attached to a common manifold. There are usually two banks, one running with all cylinders turned on (duty bank), and a reserve. In addition, there is a small emergency supply. Smaller cylinders are attached directly to the anaesthetic machine. At room temperature, nitrous oxide is a liquid within the cylinder, and while any liquid remains the pressure within the cylinder remains constant 5400 kPa (54 bar, 800 psi). When all the

Table 2.1 Medical gas cylinder colours

Gas	Old colour		New colour	
	Body	**Shoulder**	**Body**	**Shoulder**
Oxygen	Black	White	White	White
Nitrous Oxide	Blue	Blue	White	Blue
Entonox	Blue	Blue/white	White	Blue/white
Air	Grey	White/black	White	Black/white
Carbon dioxide	Grey	Grey	White	Grey
Helium/oxygen	Brown	Brown/white	White	Brown/white

liquid has evaporated, the cylinder contains only gas and as it empties, the pressure falls to zero.

Medical air

This is supplied either by a compressor or in cylinders. A compressor delivers air to a central reservoir, where it is dried and filtered to achieve the desired quality before distribution. Air is supplied to the operating theatre at 400 kPa for anaesthetic use, and at 700 kPa to power medical tools.

Vacuum

The final part of the PMGV system is medical vacuum. Two pumps are connected to a system that must be capable of generating a vacuum of at least 50 kPa below atmospheric pressure. This is delivered to the anaesthetic rooms, operating theatres and other appropriate sites. At several stages between the outlets and the pumps there are drains and bacterial filters to prevent contamination by aspirated fluids.

The anaesthetic machine

Its main functions are to:

- reduce the high pressure gases from either the pipeline or cylinders to a pressure that is safe for onward delivery to the patient;
- control the flow of gases allowing a known, accurate, and adjustable composition to be delivered into the anaesthetic breathing system.

In addition to these functions, many modern anaesthetic machines contain integral monitoring equipment and ventilators.

Reduction of pressure

Cylinders contain gases at very high pressures (see above) which can vary depending on the content or temperature of the cylinder. The gas from them first passes through reducing valves to ensure a constant supply of gas at 400 kPa is delivered to the flowmeters. As piped gases are already delivered at 400 kPa, no further pressure reduction is required.

Control of flow of gases

Traditionally, on most anaesthetic machines, this has been achieved by the use of flowmeters ('rotameters'; Fig. 2.11):

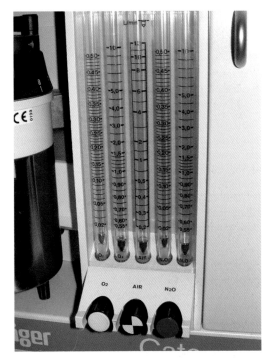

Figure 2.11 Oxygen, air and nitrous oxide flowmeters on an anaesthetic machine.

- a specific, calibrated flowmeter is used for each gas;
- a needle valve controls the flow of gas through the flowmeter;
- where accurate, low flows are required, two tubes are used in series, the first has a smaller diameter and a narrow, low flow range (e.g. 0–0.5 L/min), the second is wider with a greater flow range (0.5–10 L/min);
- a rotating bobbin floats in the gas stream, its upper edge indicating the rate of gas flow;
- several flowmeters for different gases (oxygen, air and nitrous oxide), are mounted with oxygen to the left; the control for oxygen has a different knurled finish and is usually more prominent;
- flowmeters do not regulate pressure.

Anaesthetic machines have several safety features built into the gas delivery system:

- the oxygen and nitrous oxide controls are linked preventing less than 25% oxygen from being delivered;
- an emergency oxygen 'flush' device can be used to deliver pure oxygen at greater than 40 L/min into the breathing system;

- an audible alarm to warn of failure of oxygen delivery – this discontinues the nitrous oxide supply and if the patient is breathing spontaneously air can be entrained;
- a non-return valve to minimize the effects of back-pressure on the function of flowmeters and vaporizers.

Increasingly, on many modern anaesthetic machines, flowmeters have been replaced with electronic control of gas flow. The anaesthetist simply dials in the required flow and this is delivered into the anaesthetic system. The flow of gas is then displayed on a monitor screen either numerically or as an analogue representation of a flowmeter.

The addition of anaesthetic vapours

This is achieved by the use of vaporizers, devices that produce a very accurate concentration of each inhalational anaesthetic drug (Fig. 2.12):

- Vaporizers produce a saturated vapour from a reservoir of liquid anaesthetic.

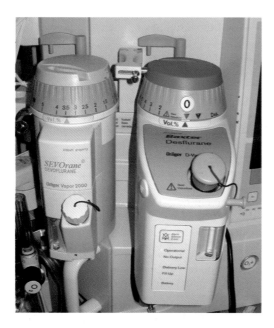

Figure 2.12 Sevoflurale vaporizer (left) and desflurane vaporizer (right) on an anaesthetic machine. Note the interlock positioned between the dials to prevent giving both vapours concurrently.

- The final concentration of anaesthetic is controlled by varying the proportion of gas passing into the vapour chamber.
- Vaporization of the anaesthetic results in loss of latent heat causing the remaining anaesthetic liquid to cool and reduces further vaporization. This would result in a fall in the concentration of anaesthetic delivered to the patient. To circumvent this problem, vaporizers incorporate a mechanism to compensate for the fall in temperature.
- Most anaesthetic machines allow more than one vaporizer to be fitted at any time. To prevent more than one vapour being given, an interlock device is fitted. This is usually a mechanical device that prevents more than one vaporizer being turned on simultaneously.

The resultant mixture of gases and vapour is finally delivered to a common outlet on the anaesthetic machine. From this point, specialized breathing systems are used to transfer the gases and vapours either to the patient or the ventilator.

Anaesthetic breathing systems

The mixture of anaesthetic gas and vapour travels from the anaesthetic machine to the patient via an anaesthetic 'circuit' or, more correctly, an anaesthetic breathing system, and finally to the patient's lungs via a facemask, laryngeal mask or tracheal tube. Historically a number of different breathing systems were used but nowadays these have largely been replaced by circle systems. The details of these systems are beyond the scope of this book but they all have a number of common features, described below. As several patients in succession may breathe through the same system, a low-resistance, disposable bacterial filter is placed at the patient end of the system, and changed between each patient to reduce the risk of cross-infection. Alternatively, disposable systems can be used, which are changed between each patient.

Components of a breathing system

All systems consist of the following:

- *A connection for fresh gas input:* usually the common gas outlet on the anaesthetic machine.

- *A reservoir bag:* Usually of 2 L capacity. This allows; the patient's peak inspiratory demands (30–40 L/min) to be met with a lower constant flow from the anaesthetic machine, manual ventilation of the patient if needed, an indication of ventilation in a spontaneously breathing patient, and acts as a further safety device, being easily distended at low pressure if obstruction occurs.
- *An adjustable expiratory valve:* To vent expired gas, helping to eliminate carbon dioxide. During spontaneous ventilation, resistance to opening is minimal so as not to impede expiration. Closing the valve allows manual ventilation by squeezing the reservoir bag.

The circle system

Many traditional anaesthetic breathing systems used high flows of gases and vapour to prevent rebreathing of expired gases and hypercarbia. The expired gas was vented to the atmosphere, thereby 'wasting' the oxygen and anaesthetic vapour it contained. The circle system (Fig. 2.13) overcomes this inefficiency by 'recycling' some of the expired gas mixture:

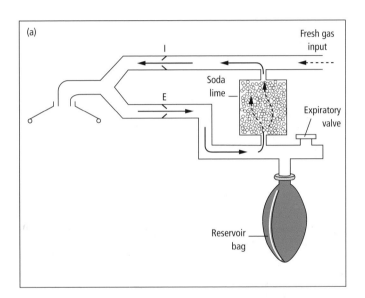

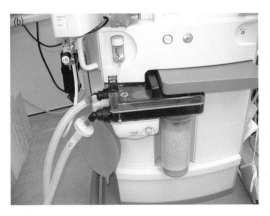

Figure 2.13 (a) Diagrammatic representation of a circle system. (I, inspiratory; E, expiratory valves). (b) Circle system on an anaesthetic machine. Most of the components shown in the diagram are integrated; only the inspiratory and expiratory tubing, the reservoir bag and soda lime container are obvious.

- the expired gases are passed through a container of soda lime (the absorber), a mixture of calcium, sodium and potassium hydroxide that removes carbon dioxide chemically;
- after the carbon dioxide has been removed the expired gas has supplementary oxygen and anaesthetic vapour added to maintain the desired concentrations, and the mixture is rebreathed by the patient;
- the gases are warmed and humidified as they pass through the absorber (a consequence of the reaction that removes carbon dioxide);
- as a result, gas flows from the anaesthetic machine can be as low as 0.3–0.5 L/min.

There are several points to note when using a circle system.

- The inspired gas is a mixture of expired and fresh gas. Its composition is affected by a number of factors including; absorption of anaesthetic by the patient and fresh gas flow. As a result, the concentration of oxygen and anaesthetic vapour within the circle does not correlate with what has been set on the vaporizer. For this reason the inspired oxygen and anaesthetic vapour concentration must be monitored to ensure that the patient is not rendered hypoxic or suffer awareness due to inadequate anaesthesia.
- An indicator is incorporated into the soda lime so that when it is unable to absorb any more carbon dioxide the granules change colour. One of the commonly used preparations changes from pink to white.

Patients can breathe spontaneously or can be ventilated via any of the anaesthetic breathing systems.

Mechanical ventilation

A wide variety of anaesthetic ventilators is available, each of which functions in a slightly different way. An outline of the principles of mechanical ventilation is given and the interested reader should consult 'further useful information' at the end of the chapter.

During spontaneous ventilation, negative intrathoracic pressure is generated, causing gas to move into the lungs. This process is reversed during mechanical ventilation. A positive pressure is applied to the anaesthetic gases to overcome airway resistance and elastic recoil of the chest, causing gas flow into the lungs.

This technique is usually referred to as *intermittent positive pressure ventilation* (IPPV). In order to generate the positive pressure, the ventilator requires a source of energy: generally gas pressure or electricity. In both spontaneous and mechanical ventilation, expiration occurs by passive recoil of the lungs and chest wall.

During mechanical ventilation the following can be controlled:

- tidal volume;
- respiratory rate;
- the mode of ventilation, usually a choice between volume and pressure controlled;
- the inspiratory and expiratory times;
- peak inspiratory pressure;
- the use of positive end expiratory pressure (PEEP).

Modes of ventilation

Anaesthetists can select the tidal volume that they want the ventilator to deliver to the patient. This is volume-controlled ventilation. It results in the generation of a pressure within the airway that is dependent on the volume set and the compliance of the patient's respiratory system. The pre-set volume will be delivered but this may result in high airway pressures and damage to the lungs (barotrauma) if there is poor respiratory compliance. The alternative is to set the maximum airway pressure generated by the ventilator; this results in a tidal volume dictated by the pressure set, and will vary depending on the patient's respiratory compliance. This is called pressure controlled ventilation (PCV) and its use reduces the risk of barotrauma, but may result in unpredictable tidal volumes with consequent hyper- or hypoventilation. A third ventilator mode found on anaesthetic machines is pressure support ventilation (PSV). This is used when the patient is breathing spontaneously but their own respiratory effort results in inadequate tidal volumes. In this case the anaesthetist can set the ventilator to detect a spontaneous breath and then provide a little positive pressure to help increase the tidal volume.

In all of these modes positive end-expiratory pressure (PEEP) can be applied to try and prevent the alveolar collapse that occurs when a patient is under general anaesthesia, improve respiratory compliance and improve ventilation/perfusion matching.

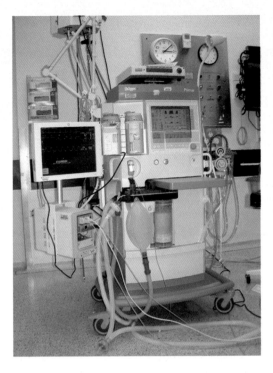

Figure 2.14 Modern integrated anaesthetic machine and monitors.

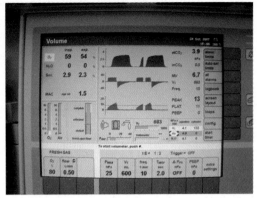

Figure 2.15 Close-up of controls and display of the anaesthetic machine in Fig. 2.14.

The modern anaesthetic machine

Advances in technology have allowed virtually all of the above functions to be integrated into a single unit (Fig. 2.14). Electronic controls (Fig. 2.15) then allow the anaesthetist to determine:

- spontaneous or controlled ventilation;
- the flow of each gas required;
- the inspired oxygen concentration.

Some machines allow the vapour concentration to be set; on others the concentration from the vaporizer is set and adjusted to achieve the required end tidal concentration. All of the above are monitored and displayed, and can be set to alarm if they fall outside predetermined limits. In case of power failure there is a back-up battery supply to maintain key operations and, if this fails, the patient can still be ventilated manually.

Minimizing theatre pollution

Unless special measures are taken, the atmosphere in the operating theatre will become polluted with anaesthetic gases. The breathing systems and mechanical ventilators described vent varying volumes of excess and expired gas into the atmosphere, the patient expires anaesthetic gas during recovery and there are leaks from anaesthetic apparatus. Although no conclusive evidence exists to link prolonged exposure to low concentrations of inhalational anaesthetics with any risks, it would seem sensible to minimize the degree of pollution within the operating theatre environment. This can be achieved in a number of ways:

- reducing the flow of gases, for example by use of a circle system;
- avoiding the use of gases, for example by use of total intravenous anaesthesia (TIVA) (see Chapter 4) or regional anaesthesia;
- using air conditioning in the theatre;
- scavenging systems.

Scavenging systems

These collect the gas vented from breathing systems and ventilators and deliver it via a pipeline system to the external atmosphere. The most widely used is an active system in which a small negative pressure is applied to the expiratory valve of the breathing system or ventilator to remove gases to the outside environment. The patient is protected against excessive negative pressure being applied to the lungs by valves with very low opening pressures. The use of such systems does not eliminate the problem of pollution; it merely shifts it from one site to another; both nitrous oxide, and to a lesser extent the inhalational anaesthetics, are potent destroyers of ozone, thereby adding to the greenhouse effect.

Intravascular cannulas

All patients undergoing anaesthesia need intravenous access in order to administer fluids, blood and drugs. There are a range of different lengths and diameters available and in general the term 'cannula' is used for those less than 7 cm in length and 'catheter' for those more than 7 cm long. The external diameter is quoted in terms of its gauge (g), and also in millimetres, and the maximum flow rate is usually quoted on the packet. The main types of cannula used are:

- Cannula over needle. The most common design, available in sizes ranging from 14 g (2.1 mm) to 24 g (0.7 mm) and colour coded according to size. They consist of a plastic cannula mounted on a metal needle with the bevel protruding. At the other end of the needle is a transparent 'flashback chamber', which can be seen to fill with blood once the needle bevel lies within the vein. All devices have a luer-lock fitting for attachment to a giving set. Some devices have 'wings' so an adhesive dressing can be used to stick it to the skin and some have a valved injection port for administering drugs. Manufacturers have developed 'safety' versions of their cannulas, which incorporate a way of covering the sharp bevel of the needle once it is removed from the cannula to prevent needlestick injuries and these are becoming increasingly popular (Fig. 2.16).
- Seldinger type. These are mainly used for central venous catheterization. Peripheral devices are available and are usually of large diameter for use when large flow rates are needed.

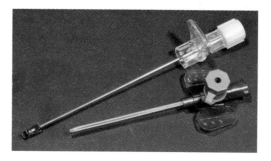

Figure 2.16 Safety cannula. Once the needle is withdrawn from the cannula, the tip is protected to reduce the risk of a needlestick injury.

Some patients may require an arterial line for close monitoring of their blood pressure (see below). There are two commonly used devices to achieve this. The first resembles a cannula-over-needle intravenous cannula except that the valved injection port is removed (to prevent mistaken intra-arterial drug injection) and replaced with a flow-switch. The second type of device is a small Seldinger cannula. Both are made of plastic, are parallel sided and in adults of 20 g diameter.

Giving sets and fluid warmers

Fluid and blood are administered to the patient from a bag hung on a drip stand through a giving set connected to the luer-lock fitting on their intravenous cannula. Different giving sets exist for different purposes; some are specifically designed to be used with certain makes of infusion pumps. In general, giving sets for intravenous fluids have a single drip chamber without a filter and narrower diameter tubing. Giving sets for use with blood and blood products have an additional drip chamber with a mesh filter to filter out any clots and wider diameter tubing.

Intravenous fluids are often at ambient temperature (20 °C), while blood and blood products may be as cold as 4 °C when given, which can lead to significant cooling of the patient; to prevent this, fluids are often warmed as they are being given. This can be achieved by passing the fluid through a section of a giving set with two concentric lumen, where the outer lumen contains a warming fluid, or by passing the fluid past heated plates. Different systems have varying maximum flow rates and varying efficiencies, but the aim is to heat the fluid being infused to as close to body temperature as possible.

Patient warming

Most patients' core temperature falls during anaesthesia as a result of exposure to a cold environment, evaporation of fluids from body cavities, being given cold intravenous fluids and breathing dry, cold anaesthetic gases. This is compounded by the loss of body temperature regulation and inability to shiver. Hypothermia is associated with delayed recovery and increased postoperative complications and must be prevented. The commonest technique used is forced air warming, a process in which warm air is blown over the surface of the patient that is not exposed for surgery via a perforated blanket (single patient use). Alternative methods are to lie the patient on a mattress heated either electrically or by perfusion with warm water.

Cell savers

These machines are used to reduce the need for allogenic blood transfusion where significant bleeding is expected, for example aortic aneurysm surgery, cardiac surgery and major orthopaedic surgery. The machine incorporates a suction unit that the surgeon uses to collect the patient's blood from the surgical field. This collected blood is then mixed with heparinized saline to prevent it clotting, passed though a filter to remove fat and other debris and then centrifuged to remove all other blood cells and leave a concentrate of red cells. These are then resuspended in solution ready for transfusion back to the patient.

Ultrasound

This uses very high-frequency sound waves emitted from a probe and reflected back from body tissues to detect changes in tissue density. A computer then interprets the reflected waves and constructs an image that can be displayed on a screen to visualize a patient's anatomy. Recently there has been increasing use of ultrasound by anaesthetists to guide needle placement during procedures such as central venous catheter insertion or peripheral nerve blocks. The aim is that keeping the needle tip under constant vision during the procedure will reduce the chance of complications and increase effectiveness of nerve blocks by better placement of local anaesthetic. Ultrasound is also increasingly being used for diagnostic purposes in trauma, for example Focused Assessment with Sonography in Trauma (FAST scanning), and in the ITU, for example to look for pleural and pericardial effusions and estimate cardiac function (filling, contractility, valve function).

Syringe pumps

There are syringe pumps available that incorporate sophisticated software that is able to predict the plasma and effect site concentrations of drugs being infused, for example propofol and remifentanil, using complicated mathematical models. The anaesthetist enters patient details such as sex, BMI, age, and the target concentration, and the syringe pump will calculate the necessary infusion rate. This is called Target Controlled Infusion (TCI). This allows for delivery of appropriate concentrations of drugs, enabling accurate titration of effect such that patients can undergo conscious sedation or Total Intravenous Anaesthesia (TIVA).

Measurement and monitoring

Measurement and monitoring are closely linked but are not synonymous. A measuring instrument becomes a monitor if it is capable of delivering a warning when the variable being measured falls outside preset limits. During anaesthesia, both the patient and the equipment being used are monitored.

Monitoring the patient

Monitoring of the ECG, blood pressure (non-invasive), pulse oximetry, capnometry, and oxygen and vapour concentrations is now regarded as essential for the safe conduct of anaesthesia. Various other parameters may also be monitored depending on the patient and the operation.

The ECG

This is easily applied and gives information on heart rate and rhythm, and may indicate the presence of ischaemia and acute disturbances of certain electrolytes (for example, potassium and calcium). It can be monitored using three leads – one applied to the right shoulder (red), another to the left shoulder (yellow) and a third to the left lower chest (green), which will give a tracing equivalent to standard lead II of the 12-lead ECG. Many ECG monitors now use five electrodes placed on the anterior chest to allow all the standard leads and V5 to be displayed. The ECG alone gives no information on the adequacy of the cardiac output and it must be remembered that it is possible to have a virtually normal ECG with minimal cardiac output.

Non-invasive blood pressure

This is the most common method of monitoring the patient's blood pressure during anaesthesia and surgery. Auscultation of the Korotkoff sounds is difficult in the operating theatre, so automated devices are widely used. A cuff, commonly placed around the arm over the brachial artery, is inflated by an electrical pump. The cuff then undergoes controlled deflation. A microprocessor-controlled pressure transducer detects variations in cuff pressure resulting from transmitted arterial pulsations. Initial pulsations represent systolic blood pressure and peak amplitude of the pulsations equates to mean arterial pressure. Diastolic is then calculated using an algorithm.

Heart rate is also determined and displayed. The pneumatic cuff must have a width that is *40% of the arm circumference* and the internal inflatable bladder should encircle at least half the arm. If the cuff is too small, the blood pressure will be overestimated, and if it is too large it will be underestimated. The frequency of blood pressure estimation can be set, and the monitor can be set to alarm if the recorded blood pressure falls outside predetermined limits. Such devices cannot measure pressure continually, and become increasingly inaccurate at extremes of pressure and in patients with an arrhythmia.

Pulse oximeter

A probe, containing a light-emitting diode (LED) and a photodetector, is applied across the tip of a digit or earlobe. The LED emits light, alternating between two different wavelengths in the visible and infrared regions of the electromagnetic spectrum. These are transmitted through the tissues and absorbed to different degrees by the tissues, oxyhaemoglobin and deoxyhaemoglobin. The intensity of light reaching the photodetector is converted to an electrical signal. Absorption by the tissues and venous blood is constant but absorption by arterial blood varies with the cardiac cycle, this allows determination of the peripheral arterial oxygen saturation (SpO_2), both as a waveform and digital reading.

Pulse oximeters are accurate to $\pm2\%$ with SpO_2 $>90\%$. The waveform can also be interpreted to give a reading of heart rate. Alarms can be set for levels of saturation and heart rate. Therefore, the pulse oximeter gives information about both the circulatory and respiratory systems and has the advantages of:

- providing continuous monitoring of oxygenation at tissue level;

- being unaffected by skin pigmentation;
- portability (mains or battery powered);
- being non-invasive.

Despite this, there are a number of important limitations of this device:

- there is failure to appreciate the severity of hypoxia; a saturation of 90% equates to a PaO_2 of 8 kPa (60 mmHg) because of the shape of the haemoglobin dissociation curve;
- it is unreliable when there is severe vasoconstriction due to the reduced pulsatile component of the signal;
- it is unreliable with certain haemoglobins:
  - carboxyhaemoglobin; results in overestimation of SaO_2;
  - methaemoglobinaemia; at an $SaO_2 > 85\%$ results in underestimation of the saturation;
- it progressively under-reads the saturation as the haemoglobin falls (but it is not affected by polycythaemia);
- it is affected by extraneous light;
- it is unreliable when there is excessive movement of the patient;
- the pulse oximeter is not an indicator of the adequacy of alveolar ventilation as hypoventilation can be compensated for by increasing the inspired oxygen concentration to maintain oxygen saturation.

In many modern anaesthetic systems the above monitors are integrated and displayed on a single screen (Fig. 2.17).

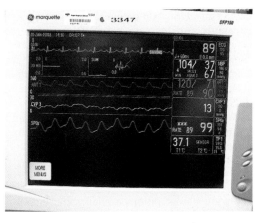

Figure 2.17 Integrated monitor displaying ECG and heart rate, non-invasive blood pressure (mmHg), arterial waveform and invasive blood pressure, central venous pressure (CVP) waveform, pulse oximeter waveform, saturation and temperature.

Capnometry

The capnometer (often referred to as a capnograph) works on the principle that carbon dioxide (CO_2) absorbs infrared light in proportion to its concentration. In a healthy person, the CO_2 concentration in air at the end of expiration ($PetCO_2$) correlates well with the partial pressure in arterial blood ($PaCO_2$), the former being lower, by 5 mmHg or 0.7 kPa. Analysis of gas in the breathing system at the end of expiration (*end-tidal CO_2 concentration*) reflects $PaCO_2$. Capnometry is primarily used as an indicator of the adequacy of ventilation; $PaCO_2$ is inversely proportional to alveolar ventilation. In patients with a low cardiac output (for example, hypovolaemia, pulmonary embolus), the gap between arterial and end-tidal carbon dioxide increases (end-tidal falls), mainly due to the development of increased areas of ventilation/perfusion mismatch. The gap also increases in patients with chest disease due to poor mixing of respiratory gases. Care must be taken in interpreting end-tidal CO_2 concentrations in these circumstances. Modern capnometers have alarms for when the end-tidal carbon dioxide is outside preset limits. Other uses of capnometry are given in Table 2.2.

Table 2.2 Uses of capnometry

- An indicator of the degree of alveolar ventilation:
  - to ensure normocapnia during mechanical ventilation
  - control the level of hypocapnia in neurosurgery
  - avoidance of hypocapnia where the cerebral circulation is impaired, e.g. in the elderly
- As a disconnection indicator (the reading suddenly falls to zero)
- To indicate that the tracheal tube is in the trachea (CO_2 in expired gas)
- As an indicator of the degree of rebreathing (presence of CO_2 in inspired gas)
- As an indicator of cardiac output. If cardiac output falls and ventilation is maintained, then end-tidal CO_2 falls as CO_2 is not delivered to the lungs, e.g.
  - hypovolaemia
  - cardiac arrest, where it can also be used to indicate effectiveness of external cardiac compression
  - massive pulmonary embolus
- It may be the first clue of the development of malignant hyperpyrexia

---

Vapour concentration analysis

Whenever a volatile anaesthetic is given the concentration in the inspired gas mixture should be monitored. This is usually achieved using infrared absorption, similar to carbon dioxide. Each volatile anaesthetic drug will absorb optimally at only one wavelength, and the degree of absorption is dependent on the volatile's concentration. A single device producing the correct wavelengths can be calibrated for all of the commonly used inhalational anaesthetics.

Peripheral nerve stimulator

This is used to assess neuromuscular blockade after giving neuromuscular blocking drugs, for example at the end of surgery, to see if the neuromuscular block has reduced sufficiently to allow for reversal. A peripheral nerve supplying a discrete muscle group is stimulated transcutaneously with a current of 50 mA. The resulting contractions are observed or measured. One arrangement is to stimulate the ulnar nerve at the wrist whilst monitoring the contractions (twitch) of the adductor pollicis. Although most often done by looking at or feeling the response, measuring either the force of contraction or the compound action potential is more objective. Sequences of stimulation used include:

- four stimuli each of 0.2 ms duration, at 2 Hz for 1.5 s, referred to as a 'train-of-four' (TOF);
- one stimulus at 50 Hz of 5 s duration – that is, a tetanic stimulus;
- two groups of three tetanic bursts at 50 Hz, 750 ms apart, called double-burst stimulation (DBS).

During non-depolarizing neuromuscular blockade, there is a *progressive* decremental response to all the sequences, termed 'fade'. In the TOF, the ratio of the amplitude of the fourth twitch (T4) to the first twitch (T1) is used as an index of the degree of neuromuscular blockade. The absence of any response is seen either with profound neuromuscular block, for example shortly after a drug has been given or is the result of failure to deliver a stimulus. During depolarizing blockade, the response to all sequences of stimulation is reduced but consistent, that is, there is no fade.

Temperature

During anaesthesia the patient's temperature should be monitored continually in accordance with recent NICE guidelines. The most commonly used device is a thermistor, a semiconductor that varies in resistance according to its temperature. This can be placed in the oesophagus (cardiac temperature) or nasopharynx (brain temperature). The rectum can be used but, apart from being unpleasant, faeces may insulate the thermistor, leading to inaccuracies. An infrared tympanic membrane thermometer can be used intermittently, but the external auditory canal must be clear. Although temperature is normally measured to help identify and prevent hypothermia, a sudden unexpected rise in a patient's temperature may be the first warning of the development of malignant hyperpyrexia (see Chapter 6).

Invasive or direct blood pressure

This is the most accurate method for measuring and monitoring blood pressure and is generally reserved for use in complex, prolonged surgery or sick patients. A cannula is inserted into a peripheral artery and connected via a fluid-filled tube to a transducer that converts the pressure signal into an electrical signal. This is then amplified and displayed as both the arterial waveform and systolic, diastolic and mean arterial blood pressure (Fig. 2.17).

Central venous pressure (CVP)

This is measured by inserting a catheter via a central vein (CVC), usually the internal jugular or subclavian, so that its tip lies at the junction of the superior vena cava and right atrium. It is then connected as described above to display a waveform and pressure (Fig. 2.17).

Although absolute values of the CVP can be measured, its trend is usually more informative. Often a 'fluid challenge' is used in the face of a low CVP. The CVP is measured, a rapid infusion of fluid is given and the change in CVP noted. In the hypovolaemic patient the CVP increases briefly and then falls back to around the previous value, whereas in the euvolaemic patient the CVP will show a greater and more sustained rise. Overtransfusion will be seen as a high, sustained CVP.

Central venous pressure is usually monitored during operations in which there is the potential for major fluid shifts, blood loss, or those patients in whom even small fluid shifts may be detrimental, for example heart failure. It is affected by a

Table 2.3   Factors affecting the central venous pressure

- The zero reference point
- Patient posture
- Fluid status
- Heart failure
- Raised intrathoracic pressure:
  - mechanical ventilation
  - coughing
  - straining
- Pulmonary embolism
- Pulmonary hypertension
- Tricuspid valve disease
- Pericardial effusion, tamponade
- Superior vena cava obstruction

variety of other factors apart from fluid balance (Table 2.3), in particular cardiac function and positive pressure ventilation. Hypotension in the presence of an elevated CVP (absolute or in response to a fluid challenge) may indicate heart failure. However, most clinicians would now accept that in these circumstances monitoring left ventricular function with either transoesophageal Doppler or one of the pulse analysis cardiac output monitoring devices is preferable.

Oesophageal Doppler cardiac output monitoring

Insertion of an oesophageal Doppler probe is relatively non-invasive, the ultrasound emitter-sensor being passed into the oesophagus to lie just behind the descending aorta, in a technique similar to that of inserting a nasogastric tube (Fig. 2.18). The underlying principle behind it is that flow through a cylinder (aorta) is proportional to its cross sectional area and the velocity of the fluid (measured using Doppler shift). Previous devices calculated the blood flow in the descending aorta and applied correction factors for upper body blood flow to calculate total cardiac output. Current devices (e.g. CardioQ-ODM^{TM}) use a nomogram incorporating age, weight and height to calibrate descending aortic blood flow velocity directly against total cardiac output, measured by thermodilation using a pulmonary artery catheter. This eliminates the need to make allowances for blood flow to the upper body which can be a significant source of error.

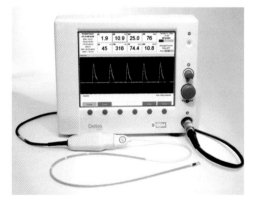

Figure 2.18 Transoesophageal Doppler monitor and oesophageal probe.

Monitoring is continuous, acute changes in cardiac output can be detected and because flow is measured in the aorta, its accuracy is not affected by changes in peripheral resistance. Optimal results require alignment of the oesophageal probe with the axial blood flow which may mean minor adjustments of the probe position. The oesophageal Doppler is a useful tool, particularly in following trends in cardiac output following fluid challenges (Fig. 2.19), and is now well established in major abdominal surgery.

Pulse analysis cardiac output monitoring

There are three systems currently available:

- PiCCO®: pulse contour continuous cardiac output monitoring. This requires a CVC and specialized arterial catheter placed in a large artery, such as the femoral artery. Calibration is performed by injecting a fixed volume of cold saline via the CVC and detecting the resulting drop in blood temperature via the arterial catheter to calculate cardiac output. Following this the arterial waveform is continually analysed and cardiac output calculated by reference to the calibration reading.
- LiDCO®: lithium dilution continuous cardiac output. This requires peripheral IV and arterial cannulas. Calibration is performed by injecting a known amount of lithium chloride through the IV cannula. The change in blood lithium concentration is measured by drawing blood from the arterial cannula past a lithium sensor and cardiac output is calculated from this. Following this, the arterial pulse pressure is continuously

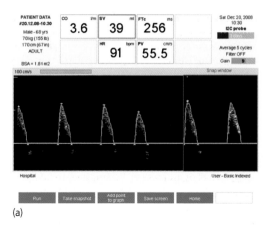

(a)

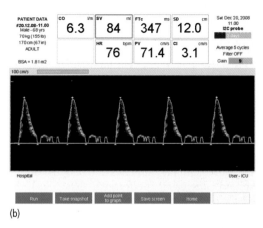

(b)

Figure 2.19 (a) Narrow waveform typical of hypovolaemia. (b) Broadening of the waveform after giving the patient an IV fluid challenge.

monitored and by reference to the calibration readings, cardiac output is derived from an algorithm that relates pulse pressure to blood flow.

Both of the above systems require regular recalibration.

- Flotrac®: this is an uncalibrated system and only requires an arterial cannula to function. This is attached to a specialized transducer and monitor that allow detailed analysis of the arterial waveform, that in turn calculates stroke volume. As pulse rate is measured, cardiac output can be calculated. The only other information required are the patient's age, sex and weight to allow compliance to be estimated. All three systems require high-quality arterial waveforms, with no damping, to allow correct evaluation of cardiac output.

Bispectral index (BIS)

This is a method for monitoring the depth of anaesthesia. General anaesthesia alters the electroencephalogram (EEG) with a general reduction in activity with increasing depth of anaesthesia. Bispectral index records the complex and difficult to interpret raw EEG data and processes it using proprietary software to produce a number between 0 (no cortical electrical activity) and 100 (fully awake) which can be used to indicate the risk of recall or awareness. When used, most operators would accept a numerical value between 40 and 60 as appropriate for general anaesthesia. Situations where BIS may be useful include when it is not possible to monitor inspired and expired volatile anaesthetic concentrations, for example cardiopulmonary bypass or TIVA, when avoidance of excessively deep anaesthesia is desirable, as in haemodynamically unstable patients, and in those at greater risk of awareness, such as those with a previous episode of awareness under general anaesthesia.

Blood loss

Strictly speaking, this is measured rather than monitored. Simple estimates of blood loss during surgery are easily performed. Swabs can be weighed, dry and wet, the increase in weight giving an indication of the amount of blood they have absorbed. The volume of blood in the suction apparatus can be measured, with allowance for irrigation fluids. Such methods are only estimates, as blood may remain in body cavities, be spilt on the floor and absorbed by drapes and gowns. In paediatric practice, where small volumes of blood loss are relatively more important, all absorbent materials are washed to remove the blood and the resultant solvent analysed by colorimetry to estimate blood loss.

Many other physiological parameters can be, and are, measured during anaesthesia when appropriate. Some examples are: clotting profiles and haemoglobin concentration in patients receiving a transfusion of a large volume of stored blood; blood glucose in diabetic patients, and arterial blood gas and acid–base analysis during the bypass phase of cardiac surgery.

It is essential to recognize that the above standards apply not only to those patients undergoing general anaesthesia, but also those receiving sedation, local or regional anaesthesia and during transfer.

Finally, one should never rely solely on monitors – regular observation and examination of the patient and clinical judgement are essential to avoid acting on false information.

Monitoring the equipment

With the increasing reliance on complex equipment to deliver anaesthesia, the AAGBI recommends that there should be continuous monitoring of the continuity of the oxygen supply and correct functioning of the breathing system.

Oxygen supply

All anaesthetic machines are fitted with a device warning of oxygen supply failure. Continuous monitoring of the oxygen concentration in the inspired gas mixture is considered essential. This is usually achieved using a fuel-cell oxygen analyser that produces a current proportional to the oxygen concentration, displayed as a numeric value of oxygen concentration. *It must be remembered that the inspired oxygen concentration does not guarantee adequate arterial oxygen saturation* as it may be insufficient to compensate for the effects of hypoventilation and ventilation/perfusion mismatch (see Chapter 7).

Breathing systems

Irrespective of whether the patient is breathing spontaneously or being ventilated, capnometry will alert the anaesthetist to most of the common problems, e.g. disconnection (loss of reading), exhaustion of the CO_2 absorber (failure of the reading to fall to zero during inspiration), inadequate gas flow (increased *end-tidal CO_2* although hypoxia is a greater risk), hyper/hypoventilation (decreased/increased *end-tidal CO_2*, respectively). In addition, when a patient is mechanically ventilated, airway pressures must be monitored to avoid excessive pressures being generated within the lungs. Airway pressure monitoring can also be used as a secondary indicator of inadequate ventilation in ventilated patients; high pressures may be the result of obstruction (for example, blocked tracheal tube, bronchospasm), and loss of pressure may be the result of a disconnection. The latter function may be specifically used as a 'disconnection alarm'.

📖 FURTHER USEFUL INFORMATION

Aitkenhead A, Rowbotham DJ, Smith G (eds). *Textbook of anaesthesia*, 5th edn. Edinburgh: Churchill Livingstone, 2006.

Al-Shaikh B, Stacey S. *Essentials of anaesthetic equipment*, 3rd edn. Edinburgh: Churchill Livingstone, 2007.

Cook T, Howes B. Supraglottic airway devices: recent advances. Continuing Education in Anaesthesia, Critical Care and Pain. 2011;11 (2):56–61

[An article explaining the numerous variation of the 'classic LMA' and their uses and pitfalls.]

McGuire B, Younger R. Rigid indirect laryngoscopy and optical stylets. Continuing Education in Anaesthesia, Critical Care and Pain. 2010;10:48–51.

Yentis SM, Hirsch NP, Smith GB. *Anaesthesia and intensive care A to Z: an encyclopaedia of principles and practice.* Edinburgh: Butterworth Heinemann, 2003.

http://www.theairwaysite.com/pages/page_content/airway_equipment.aspx
[This site is aimed at emergency physicians and orientated to American practice. It does, however, contain some useful information about airway equipment.]

www.lmaco.com/
[The laryngeal mask airway company website, which has instruction manuals for all the variations in current use. Note that several other companies now make laryngeal mask-type devices.]

http://www.capnography.com/index.html
[This is an excellent site if you want to know more about capnography. Very detailed, so be warned.]

http://www.mhra.gov.uk/
[Medicines and Healthcare products Regulatory Agency (UK) ensures that medicines, healthcare products and medical equipment meet appropriate standards of safety, quality, performance and effectiveness, and are used safely. Report adverse events to this agency in the UK.]

http://www.frca.co.uk/
[Anaesthesia UK. The most popular website for trainees in anaesthesia.]

All websites last accessed February 2012.

> **?** **SELF-ASSESSMENT**
>
> **Short-answer questions**
>
> 2.1 Describe briefly the physical principles of a pulse oximeter. What circumstances limit the usefulness of this device?
>
> 2.2 Describe how oxygen, nitrous oxide and medical air are stored and supplied to the operating theatres. What are the key safety characteristics of the hoses carrying these gases in the operating theatre?
>
> 2.3 What are the key functions performed by an anaesthesia machine?
>
> 2.4 How do you size a non-invasive blood pressure cuff? Why is it important to use the correct size? Briefly describe the principles of how an automated NIBP machine works.
>
> **True/false questions**
>
> 2.1 When using a circle anaesthetic breathing system:
>   a carbon dioxide (CO_2) from the patient is flushed into the atmosphere to prevent it being rebreathed;
>   b some of the gas expired by the patient is rebreathed;
>   c the setting on the vaporizer indicates the concentration of vapour in the circle;
>   d the patient cannot be allowed to breathe spontaneously.
>
> 2.2 A pulse oximeter:
>   a is highly accurate at all readings of SpO_2;
>   b gives a reliable indication of ventilation;
>   c gives a reliable indication of tissue oxygenation;
>   d is reliable with all forms of haemoglobin.
>
> 2.3 A capnometer:
>   a works on the principle that carbon dioxide absorbs ultraviolet light;
>   b gives the same reading as the $PaCO_2$;
>   c gives an indication of the adequacy of ventilation;
>   d remains reliable in low cardiac output states (for example, hypovolaemia).
>
> 2.4 With regard to medical gases:
>   a oxygen is supplied to the anaesthetic machine by the piped system at a pressure of 4000 kPa;
>   b the pipeline carrying nitrous oxide (N_2O) is coloured white;
>   c the flowmeters (rotameters) on the anaesthetic machine reduce the pressure of gas supplied to the patient;
>   d nitrous oxide in a full cylinder is present as a liquid.
>
> 2.5 Supra-glottic airway devices:
>   a will prevent aspiration of gastric contents;
>   b are only suitable for use in spontaneously breathing patients;
>   c have a moulded gel cuff to provide a laryngeal seal;
>   d can only be used in adults.

Drugs and fluids used during anaesthesia

Anaesthetists have to be familiar with a wide range of drugs – those directly associated with anaesthesia, and also medications that may impact upon anaesthesia. Furthermore, unlike in most other branches of medicine, drugs associated with anaesthesia are almost always given parenterally, either intravenously or via inhalation, usually produce profound physiological changes, and often have serious undesirable actions in addition to their intended effects. As well as drugs, many patients will also require intravenous fluids, blood, and blood products during anaesthesia, surgery, and postoperatively.

Premedication

This refers to any drugs given in the period before induction of anaesthesia, in addition to those normally taken by the patient. Some drugs are given with specific intentions.

Modification of pH and volume of gastric contents

Patients are starved preoperatively to reduce the risk of regurgitation and aspiration of gastric acid at the induction of anaesthesia (see below). However, certain high-risk groups may be given specific therapy to try to increase the pH and reduce the volume of gastric contents:

- women who are pregnant, particularly in the later stages of pregnancy;
- patients who require emergency surgery;.
- patients with a hiatus hernia, who are at an increased risk of regurgitation;
- patients who are morbidly obese.

Clinical Anaesthesia Lecture Notes, Fourth Edition. Carl Gwinnutt and Matthew Gwinnutt.
© 2012 John Wiley & Sons, Ltd. Published 2012 by John Wiley & Sons, Ltd.

A variety of drug combinations are used to try and increase the pH and reduce the volume of gastric contents:

- *ranitidine (H$_2$ antagonist)*: 150 mg orally 12 hours and 2 hours preoperatively;
- *omeprazole (proton pump inhibitor)*: 40 mg 3–4 hours preoperatively;
- *metoclopramide*: 10 mg orally preoperatively – it increases both gastric emptying and lower oesophageal sphincter tone and is often given in conjunction with ranitidine;
- *oral sodium citrate (0.3 M)*: 30 mL orally to chemically neutralize residual acid; it is most commonly used immediately before induction of anaesthesia for caesarean section.

If a naso- or orogastric tube is in place, this can be used to aspirate gastric contents.

Analgesia

There has been interest in giving preoperative analgesia to patients who are not in pain prior to surgery, so called pre-emptive analgesia. It is known that tissue damage during surgery leads to an increased sensitivity of pain-conduction pathways in the peripheral and central nervous system. This up-regulation makes postoperative pain more severe and can lead to chronic pain problems. The aim is that giving analgesia before the surgical tissue damage will stop the sensitization resulting in reduced postoperative pain, which is easier to treat, and prevent chronic pain. So far this approach has not shown a proven benefit.

Patients are sometimes also given oral analgesia (paracetamol or NSAIDs) prior to short daycase procedures, for example knee arthroscopy and cytoscopy simply to give enough time for it to have its effect by the end of the operation.

Anti-emetics

These drugs are often given as a premed to try and reduce the incidence of postoperative nausea and vomiting (PONV). However, there is increasing evidence that they are more effective if given during or at the end of anaesthesia (see below).

Miscellaneous

A variety of other drugs are commonly given prophylactically before anaesthesia and surgery, for example:

- *steroids*: to patients on long-term treatment, or who have received them within the past 3 months;
- *antibiotics*: to patients with prosthetic or diseased heart valves or undergoing joint replacement or bowel surgery;
- *anticoagulants*: as prophylaxis against deep venous thrombosis;
- *transdermal glyceryl trinitrate (GTN)* as patches for patients with ischaemic heart disease to reduce the risk of coronary ischaemia;
- *eutectic mixture of local anaesthetics (EMLA)*: a topically applied local anaesthetic cream to reduce the pain of inserting an IV cannula.

> The majority of the patient's own regular medications should be taken as normal, unless instructed otherwise by the anaesthetist.

Intravenous anaesthetic drugs

This group of drugs is most commonly used to induce anaesthesia. After intravenous (IV) injection, these drugs are carried in the bloodstream into the cerebral circulation. As they are very lipid soluble, they quickly cross the blood-brain barrier, resulting in loss of consciousness. Subsequently the drug is rapidly redistributed to other tissues (initially the muscles and then fat), and so the plasma and brain concentrations fall and the patient recovers consciousness. A single bolus of these drugs has a rapid onset, short duration of action with rapid recovery. Despite this, complete elimination of some drugs, usually by hepatic metabolism, takes much longer and repeated doses may lead to accumulation and delayed recovery. This is seen typically with thiopental and currently the only exception to this is propofol (see below). All these drugs cause depression of the cardiovascular and respiratory systems. The dose required to induce anaesthesia is significantly reduced in those patients who are elderly, frail, hypovolaemic or have compromise of their cardiovascular system. A synopsis of the drugs commonly used is given in Table 3.1.

Table 3.1 Intravenous drugs used for the induction of anaesthesia and their effects

Drug CNS	Induction dose (mg/kg)	Speed of induction (s)	Duration of action (min)	Effects on CVS	Effects on RS	Effects on CNS	Other side-effects	Comments
Propofol	1.5–2.5	30–45	4–7	Hypotension, worse if hypovolaemic or cardiac disease	Apnoea up to 60s, depression of ventilation	Decreases CBF and ICP	Pain on injection, involuntary movement, hiccoughs	Non-cumulative, repeated injections or infusion used to maintain anaesthesia (see TIVA)
Etomidate	0.2–0.3	30–40	3–6	Relatively less cardiovascular depression	Depression of ventilation	Decreases CBF and ICP, anticonvulsant	Pain on injection, involuntary movement, hiccoughs	Emulsion available, less painful. No histamine release, non-cumulative, suppresses steroid synthesis
Thiopental	2–6	20–30	9–10	Dose dependent hypotension, worse if hypovolaemic or cardiac disease	Apnoea, depression of ventilation	Decreases CBF and ICP, anticonvulsant	Rare but severe adverse reactions	Patients may 'taste' garlic or onions! Cumulative, delayed recovery after repeat doses
Ketamine	1–2	50–70	10–12	Minimal in fit patients, better tolerated if cardiovascular compromise	Minimal depression of ventilation, laryngeal reflexes better preserved, bronchodilation	CBF maintained, profound analgesia	Vivid hallucinations	Subanaesthetic doses cause analgesia. Can be used as sole anaesthetic drug in adverse circumstances, e.g. prehospital
Midazolam	0.1–0.3	40–70	10–15	Dose dependent hypotension, worse if hypovolaemic or cardiac disease	Depression of ventilation, worse in elderly	Mildly anticonvulsant		Causes amnesia

CVS: cardiovascular system; RS: respiratory system; CNS: central nervous system; CBF: cerebral blood flow; ICP: intracranial pressure; TIVA: total intravenous anaesthesia.

Inhaled anaesthetic drugs

Although these drugs can be used to induce anaesthesia, they are most commonly used to maintain anaesthesia. Apart from nitrous oxide (N_2O), they are halogenated hydrocarbons. They all have relatively low boiling points, so they evaporate easily at ambient temperature and hence are often referred to as vapours. A controlled amount of the vapour that is produced is added to the fresh gas flow (oxygen and air or nitrous oxide) and breathed by the patient. Once in the lungs the vapour diffuses into the pulmonary capillary blood and is distributed via the systemic circulation to the brain and other tissues. The depth of anaesthesia produced is directly related to the partial pressure that the vapour exerts in the brain, and this is closely related to the partial pressure in the alveoli. The rate at which the alveolar partial pressure can be changed determines the rate of change in the brain and hence the speed of, induction, change in depth, and recovery from anaesthesia. Even the most rapid induction using these drugs takes several minutes to achieve the same depth of anaesthesia that is achieved within seconds of giving an IV anaesthetic drug. The inspired concentration of all of these compounds is expressed as the percentage by volume. All the inhalational anaesthetics cause dose-dependent depression of the cardiovascular and respiratory systems. A synopsis of the currently used drugs used is given in Table 3.2.

There are two concepts that will help in understanding the use of inhalational anaesthetics: solubility and minimum alveolar concentration (MAC).

Solubility

The rate of change of depth of anaesthesia is determined by how quickly the alveolar, and hence brain, partial pressure of anaesthetic can be altered. One of the main factors governing alveolar partial pressure for a given inhalational anaesthetic is its solubility in blood. One that is relatively *soluble* in blood (for example, isoflurane) will dissolve readily in the plasma and not exert a very high partial pressure. Consequently, a relatively large amount of the anaesthetic has to diffuse from the alveoli before the partial pressure in the blood and the brain begins to rise. Conversely, if an agent is *insoluble* in blood (for example, desflurane), only a small amount has to diffuse from the alveoli into the blood to cause a rise blood and brain partial pressure and therefore an increase in depth of anaesthesia can be achieved more quickly. Reducing the depth or recovery from anaesthesia follows similar principles in reverse; a greater amount of a soluble agent will have to be excreted for the brain, blood and alveolar partial pressure to fall, which takes proportionately longer.

Table 3.2 Inhalational anaesthetic drugs and their effects

Compound	MAC in oxygen/ air	Solubility	Effect on CVS	Effect on RS	Effect on CNS	Comments
Sevoflurane	2.2%	Low; rapid changes of depth	↓ BP, vasodilatation	Depresses ventilation	Minimal effect on CBF at clinical concentration	Popular for inhalation induction
Desflurane	6.0%	Low; rapid changes of depth	↓ BP, ↑ HR	Depresses ventilation	Minimal effect on CBF at clinical concentration	Pungent, boils at 23 °C
Isoflurane	1.3%	Medium	↓ BP, ↑ HR, vasodilatation	Depresses ventilation	Slight ↑ CBF and ICP	Pungency limits use for induction

MAC: minimum alveolar concentration; CVS: cardiovascular system; RS: respiratory system; CNS: central nervous system; BP: blood pressure; HR: heart rate; CBF: cerebral blood flow; ICP: intracranial pressure; ECG: electroencephalograph.

Other factors that determine the speed at which the alveolar concentration rises include:

- *A high inspired concentration*, limited clinically by the degree of irritation caused by the vapour.
- *Alveolar ventilation*. This is most pronounced for drugs with a high solubility. As large amounts are removed from the alveoli, increasing ventilation ensures more rapid replacement.
- *Cardiac output*: If high, this results in a greater pulmonary blood flow, increasing uptake and thereby lowering the alveolar partial pressure. If low, the converse occurs and the alveolar concentration rises more rapidly.

Minimum alveolar concentration

To compare the potencies and side effects of the inhalational anaesthetics the concept of *minimum alveolar concentration* (MAC) is used. Minimum alveolar concentration is the concentration required to prevent movement following a surgical stimulus in 50% of subjects. At 1 MAC, or multiples thereof, the anaesthetic effect of different drugs will be the same and a comparison of the side-effects can be made. Compounds with a low potency (such as desflurane) will have a high MAC; those with a high potency (such as isoflurane) will have a low MAC.

Table 3.3 **Factors affecting the minimum alveolar concentration (MAC) of inhalational anaesthetic drugs**

Increasing MAC	Decreasing MAC
• Infants, children	• Neonates, elderly
• Hyperthermia	• Hypothermia
• Hyperthyroidism	• Hypothyroidism
• Hypernatraemia	• Hyponatraemia
• Chronic alcohol intake	• Acute alcohol intake
• Chronic opioid use	• Acute intake of opioids, benzodiazepines, TCAs, clonidine
• Increased catecholamines	• Lithium, magnesium
	• Pregnancy
	• Anaemia

TCAs: tricyclic antidepressants

The effects of inhalational anaesthetics are additive, therefore two values for MAC are often quoted – the value in oxygen (Table 3.2) and the value when given with a stated percentage of nitrous oxide (which has its own MAC), which will clearly be less. The value of MAC is also affected by a number of other patient factors (Table 3.3).

Nitrous oxide

Nitrous oxide (N_2O) is a colourless, sweet-smelling, non-irritant vapour with moderate analgesic properties but low anaesthetic potency (MAC 105%). The maximum safe inspired concentration that can be administered without the risk of causing hypoxia is approximately 70%, therefore unconsciousness or anaesthesia sufficient to allow surgery is rarely achieved. Consequently, it is usually given in conjunction with one of the other vapours. Nitrous oxide is available in cylinders premixed with oxygen as a 50:50 mixture called 'Entonox', which is used as an analgesic in obstetrics and by the emergency services.

Systemic effects

- Cardiovascular depression, worse in patients with pre-existing cardiac disease.
- Slight increase in the respiratory rate and a decrease in the tidal volume. It decreases the ventilatory response to hypercarbia and hypoxia.
- Cerebral vasodilatation, increasing intracranial pressure (ICP).
- Diffuses into air-filled cavities more rapidly than nitrogen can escape, causing either a rise in pressure (for example, in the middle ear) or an increase in volume (for example, within the gut or an air embolus).
- May cause bone-marrow suppression by inhibiting the production of factors necessary for the synthesis of DNA. The length of exposure necessary may be as short as a few hours, and recovery usually occurs within 1 week.
- At the end of anaesthesia, nitrous oxide rapidly diffuses into the alveoli reducing the partial pressure of oxygen and can result in hypoxia (diffusion hypoxia) if the patient is breathing air. This can be overcome by increasing the inspired oxygen concentration during recovery from anaesthesia.

Total intravenous anaesthesia

When IV drugs alone are given to induce and maintain anaesthesia, the term 'total intravenous anaesthesia' (TIVA) is used. For a drug to be of use in maintaining anaesthesia, it must be rapidly metabolized to inactive substances or eliminated to prevent accumulation and delayed recovery, and must have no unpleasant side effects. Currently, an infusion of propofol is the only technique used; ketamine is associated with an unpleasant recovery, etomidate suppresses steroid synthesis, and recovery after barbiturates is prolonged due to their accumulation (see Chapter 4).

Neuromuscular blocking drugs

These work by preventing acetylcholine interacting with the postsynaptic (nicotinic) receptors on the motor end plate on the skeletal muscle membrane (and possibly other sites). Muscle relaxants are divided into two groups and named to reflect what is thought to be their mode of action.

Depolarizing neuromuscular blocking drugs

Suxamethonium

This is the only drug of this type in regular clinical use. It comes ready prepared (50 mg/mL, 2 mL ampoules). The dose in adults is 1.5 mg/kg IV. After injection, there is a short period of muscle fasciculation as the muscle membrane is depolarized, followed by muscular paralysis in 40–60 s. Recovery occurs spontaneously as suxamethonium is hydrolysed by the enzyme plasma (pseudo-) cholinesterase, and normal neuromuscular transmission is restored after 4–6 min. This rapid onset makes it the drug of choice to facilitate tracheal intubation in patients likely to regurgitate and aspirate, as part of a technique called a rapid sequence induction (RSI, see Chapter 6).

Suxamethonium has no direct effect on the cardiovascular, respiratory, or central nervous systems. Bradycardia secondary to vagal stimulation

Table 3.4 Important side effects of suxamethonium

- Malignant hyperpyrexia in susceptible patients
- Increased intraocular pressure which may cause loss of vitreous in penetrating eye injuries
- Muscular pain around the limb girdles, most common 24 h after administration in young adults
- Histamine release: usually localized but may cause an anaphylactic reaction
- Prolonged apnoea in patients with pseudocholinesterase deficiency (see below)
- A predictable rise in serum potassium by 0.5–0.7 mmol/L in all patients
- A massive rise in serum potassium may provoke arrhythmias in patients with:
  - burns, maximal 3 weeks to 3 months after the burn
  - denervation injury, e.g. spinal cord trauma, maximal after 1 week
  - muscle dystrophies, e.g. Duchenne's
  - crush injury

is common after very large or repeated doses, and can be avoided by pretreatment with atropine. Suxamethonium has a number of important side effects (Table 3.4).

Pseudocholinesterase deficiency

A variety of genes have been identified that are involved in plasma cholinesterase production, some of which lead to altered metabolism of suxamethonium. The most significant genotypes are:

- normal homozygotes: sufficient enzyme activity to hydrolyse suxamethonium in 4–6 min (950 per 1000 population);
- atypical heterozygotes: slightly reduced enzyme activity levels; suxamethonium lasts 10–20 min (50 per 1000);
- atypical homozygotes: marked deficiency of active enzyme; members of this group remain apnoeic for up to 2 hours after being given suxamethonium (<1 per 1000).

Treatment of a patient found to have severe deficiency of pseudocholinesterase is with maintenance of anaesthesia or sedation and ventilatory support until spontaneous recovery occurs. The patient should subsequently be warned and given a card that carries details and, because of its inherited nature, the remainder of the family should be investigated.

Non-depolarizing neuromuscular blocking drugs

These drugs compete with acetylcholine and block its access to the postsynaptic receptor sites on the muscle but do not cause depolarization. (They may also block pre-synaptic receptors responsible for facilitating the release of acetylcholine.) The time to maximum effect, that is when relaxation is adequate to allow tracheal intubation, is relatively slow compared with suxamethonium, generally 1.5–3 min. A synopsis of the drugs used is given in Table 3.5.

They are used in two ways:

- following suxamethonium to maintain muscle relaxation during surgery;
- to facilitate tracheal intubation in non-urgent situations.

Although recovery of normal neuromuscular function will eventually occur spontaneously after the use of these drugs, it is often accelerated by the administration of an anticholinesterase (see below).

Anticholinesterases

The action of all the neuromuscular blocking drugs will wear off spontaneously with time but this is not always clinically appropriate or

Table 3.5 Non depolarizing neuromuscular blocking drugs

Drug	Dose for intubation	Maintenance dose	Time to intubation (s)	Clinical duration of action (min)	Systemic effects	Comments
Atracurium	0.5–0.6 mg/kg	0.15–0.2 mg/kg; 30–50 mg/h infusion	90–120	40	Cutaneous histamine release, ↓ BP	Spontaneous degradation in plasma.
Cisatracurium	0.1–0.15 mg/kg	0.03 mg/kg; 6–12 mg/h infusion	120–150	50	Minimal	Single isomer of atracurium. Greater potency, longer duration of action. Minimal histamine release.
Rocuronium	0.6–0.7 mg/kg For RSI 1.0–1.2 mg/kg	0.15–0.2 mg/kg; 30–50 mg/h infusion	60–90 after 0.6 mg/kg, 40–50 after 1.2 mg/kg	30–40 60–70	Minimal	Alternative to suxamethonium for RSI
Vecuronium	0.1 mg/kg	0.02–0.03 mg/kg; 6–10 mg/h infusion	120–150	30–35	Minimal, no histamine release	White powder, dissolved before use
Mivacurium	0.15–0.2 mg/kg	0.1 mg/kg	150–180	15–20	Histamine released if large dose injected rapidly	Metabolized by plasma cholinesterase. Rapid recovery, reversal often unnecessary
Pancuronium	0.1 mg/kg	0.015 mg/kg	150–180	60–75	↑ BP, ↑ HR	Long-acting

BP: blood pressure; HR: heart rate; RSI: rapid sequence induction.

convenient. If reversal of neuromuscular blockade due to a non-depolarizing neuromuscular blocker is required, an anticholinesterase is given (they cannot reverse the blockade induced by suxamethonium and would actually potentiate its action!). This inhibits the action of the enzyme acetylcholinesterase, leading to an increase in the concentration of acetylcholine within the synaptic cleft of the neuromuscular junction. It is accepted practice that anticholinesterases are only used once there is return of at least two twitches on peripheral nerve stimulation using the train-of-four assessment (see Chapter 2). If used in the presence of more profound neuromuscular block there is an increased chance of residual muscle paralysis in the immediate postoperative period.

Anticholinesterases also increase the amount of acetylcholine within parasympathetic synapses (muscarinic receptors), causing bradycardia, spasm of the bowel, bladder and bronchi, increased bronchial secretions, etc. To prevent these unwanted muscarinic effects they are always administered with a suitable dose of an anti-muscarinic.

The most commonly used anticholinesterase is neostigmine:

- a fixed dose of 2.5 mg intravenously is used in adults;
- its maximal effect is seen after approximately 5 min and lasts for 20–30 min;
- it is given concurrently with either atropine 1.2 mg or glycopyrrolate 0.5 mg.

Sugammadex

This is a relatively new drug that is able to reverse any intensity of neuromuscular block induced by drugs of the aminosteroid group, i.e. rocuronium and vecuronium. The dose needed, and time taken, for complete return of neuromuscular function vary depending on the intensity of the neuromuscular block to be reversed and range from 4–16 mg/kg and 1–3 min. Sugammadex is a doughnut-shaped molecule that surrounds a molecule of neuromuscular blocker in the plasma, rendering it inactive. The sugammadex-muscle relaxant complexes are then excreted in the urine. Using sugammadex removes the need for, and unwanted side-effects of, both anticholinesterases and antimuscarinics when reversing residual neuromuscular block. At present, it is not used routinely for reversal of neuromuscular blockade

due to its cost, but it is used for reversal of rocuronium-induced neuromuscular blockade in an emergency such as 'can't intubate, can't ventilate' (see below).

Analgesic drugs

Analgesic drugs are used as part of the anaesthetic technique to reduce the autonomic response to surgery, allow lower concentrations of inhalational or intravenous drugs to be given to maintain anaesthesia, and to try to minimize immediate postoperative pain.

Opioid analgesics

This term is used to describe all drugs that have an analgesic effect mediated through opioid receptors including both naturally occurring and synthetic compounds. The term 'opiate' is reserved for naturally occurring substances, such as morphine. They produce their effects at a cellular level by activating opioid receptors. These receptors are distributed throughout the central nervous system, in particular in the substantia gelatinosa of the spinal cord and the peri-aqueductal grey matter of the mid-brain. There are several types of opioid receptors and since their identification they have had a variety of names. The current nomenclature for identification of opioid receptors is that approved by the International Union of Pharmacology: MOP, KOP, DOP and NOP receptors (previously called mu, kappa and delta opioid peptide, NOP has no previous name), each of which has a number of different subtypes. Opioid analgesics can have pure agonist, partial agonist or mixed (agonist and antagonist) actions at the receptors.

Pure agonists

This group of drugs produces the classical effects of opioids: analgesia, euphoria, sedation, depression of ventilation and physical dependence. The systemic effects of opioids are due to both central and peripheral actions and are summarized in Table 3.6.

A synopsis of the pure agonists used in anaesthesia is given in Table 3.7. Because of the potential for physical dependence, there are strict rules laid out in the Misuse of Drugs Act 1971 which govern the issue and use of most opioid drugs (see below).

Table 3.6 Central and peripheral effects of opioids

Central nervous system	Respiratory system	Gastrointestinal tract
Analgesia Sedation Euphoria Nausea and vomiting Pupillary constriction	Antitussive Bronchospasm in susceptible patients	Reduced peristalsis causing: • constipation • delayed gastric emptying Constriction of sphincters
Depression of ventilation: • rate more than depth • reduced response to carbon dioxide	**Cardiovascular system**	**Endocrine system**
Depression of vasomotor centre Addiction (not with normal clinical use)	Peripheral venodilatation Bradycardia due to vagal stimulation	Release of ADH and catecholamines
	Urinary tract	**Skin**
	Increased sphincter tone and urinary retention	Itching

ADH: antidiuretic hormone.

Table 3.7 The pure opioid agonists used in anaesthesia

Drug	Route given	Dose	Speed of onset	Duration of action (min)	Comments
Morphine	IM	0.2–0.3 mg/kg	20–30 min	60–120	Also given subcutaneously, rectally, epidurally, intrathecally
	IV	0.1–0.15 mg/kg	5–10 min	45–60	Effective against visceral pain and pain of myocardial ischaemia. Less effective in trauma
Fentanyl	IV	1–3 mcg/kg	2–3 min	20–30	Short procedures, spontaneous ventilation
		5–10 mcg/kg	1–2 min	30–60	Long procedures, controlled ventilation
Alfentanil	IV	10 mcg/kg	30–60 s	5–10	Short procedures. May cause profound respiratory depression
	IV infusion	0.5–2 mcg/kg/min	30–60 s	Infusion dependent	Long procedures, controlled ventilation
Remifentanil	IV infusion	0.1–0.3 mcg/kg/min	15–30 s	Infusion dependent	Major procedures. Very rapid recovery. Profound respiratory depression. Widely used in TIVA
Pethidine	IM	1–2 mg/kg	15–20 min	30–60	Marked nausea and vomiting. Less effect on smooth muscle

TIVA: total intravenous anaesthesia.

Tramadol

A weak agonist predominantly at MOP receptors with approximately 10% of morphine's potency, but it is not a controlled drug. It causes the same side effects as morphine, however in equi-analgesic doses the respiratory depression and constipation are less severe. Tramadol also blocks the reuptake of noradrenaline and 5-HT within the CNS, thereby augmenting descending inhibitory pathways that modulate pain perception. As a result, naloxone can only reverse the MOP receptor mediated actions, providing only partial reversal. Well absorbed orally, the dose is 50–100 mg not more frequently than 4 hourly. Similar doses can be given IV or IM.

Buprenorphine

This is a partial agonist, but 30 times more potent than morphine, with a longer duration of action, up to 8 hours. It is well absorbed when given sublingually. Nausea and vomiting may be severe and prolonged. Not completely reversed by naloxone (see below).

The pure antagonist

The only one in common clinical use is naloxone. This has antagonist actions at all the opioid receptors, reversing all the centrally mediated effects of pure opioid agonists:

- the initial IV dose in adults is 0.1–0.4 mg, effective in less than 60 s and lasts 30–45 min;
- it has a limited effect against opioids, with partial or mixed actions, and complete reversal may require very high (10 mg) doses;
- following a severe overdose, either accidental or deliberate, several doses or an infusion of naloxone may be required, as its duration of action is shorter than most opioids;
- interestingly, naloxone also reverses the analgesia produced by acupuncture, suggesting that this is probably mediated in part by the release of endogenous opioids.

The regulation of opioid drugs

Some drugs have the potential for abuse and to cause physical dependence, and their use in medicine is carefully regulated. The Misuse of Drugs Act 1971 relates to 'dangerous or otherwise harmful drugs', which are designated 'controlled drugs' and includes the opioids. The Act attempts to prevent the misuse of these substances by imposing a total prohibition on their manufacture, possession, and supply. The Misuse of Drugs Regulations 2001 permits the use of controlled drugs in medicine. The drugs covered by these regulations are classified into five schedules, each subject to a different level of control:

Schedule 1: hallucinogenic drugs, including cannabis and lysergic acid diethylamide (LSD), which currently have no recognized therapeutic use;
Schedule 2: this includes opioids, major stimulants (amphetamines and cocaine);
Schedule 3: drugs thought less likely to be misused than those in schedule 2, and includes barbiturates, minor stimulants, buprenorphine, and temazepam;
Schedule 4: this is split into two parts:
  ○ benzodiazepines (except temazepam), ketamine, which are recognized as having the potential for abuse
  ○ androgenic steroids, clenbuterol and growth hormones.
Schedule 5: Preparations which contain very low concentrations of codeine or morphine, such as cough mixtures.

Supply and custody of schedule 2 drugs

In the operating theatre complex, these drugs are supplied by the pharmacy, usually at the signed, written request of a senior member of the nursing staff, specifying the drug and total quantity required. These drugs must be stored in a locked safe, cabinet, or room, constructed and maintained in a way that prevents unauthorized access. A record must be kept of their use in the 'Controlled Drugs Register' and must comply with the following requirements:

- separate parts of the register can be used for different drugs or strengths of drugs within a single class;
- the class of drug must be recorded at the head of each page;
- entries must be in chronological sequence;
- entries must be made on the day of the transaction or the next day;
- entries must be in ink or otherwise indelible;
- no cancellation, alteration or obliteration may be made;
- corrections must be accompanied by a dated footnote;
- the register must not be used for any other purpose;
- a separate register may be used for each department (each theatre);
- registers must be kept for two years after the last dated entry.

The specific details required with respect to supply of controlled drugs (for the patient) are: the date of the transaction, name of person supplied (the patient's name), license of person to be in possession (doctor's signature with name printed), amount given to the patient and the amount, if any from the ampoule, not given and destroyed. A fresh ampoule(s) must be used for each patient.

Non-steroidal anti-inflammatory drugs (NSAIDs)

These drugs inhibit the enzyme cyclo-oxygenase (COX) therefore preventing the synthesis of prostaglandins, prostacyclins and thromboxane A2 from arachidonic acids. They have anti-inflammatory, analgesic, antipyretic actions. There are two main iso-enzymes of cyclo-oxygenase, COX-1, COX-2:

- *COX-1*: constitutive enzyme, responsible for synthesizing prostaglandins involved in protection of the integrity of the gastric mucosa, maintenance of renal blood flow, particularly during shock, platelet aggregation to reduce bleeding, and bone healing.
- *COX-2*: inducible, peripherally by surgery, trauma, endotoxins, and in the central nervous system (CNS) by pain.

The inhibition of COX-1 produces the unwanted effects, inhibition of COX-2 the desired therapeutic effects. The older NSAIDs are non-specific and associated with a greater incidence of complications with elderly patients being particularly vulnerable. More recently, COX-2 specific NSAIDs have become available. These target only the inducible form of the enzyme and were originally thought to have a lower incidence of complications. Unfortunately in long-term clinical use this does not appear to be the case and some of these drugs have been associated with increased risk of stroke and myocardial infarction. Their main role now is in the short term management of acute pain. The relative and absolute contraindications to the use of these drugs are given in Table 3.8.

A commonly used NSAID in the perioperative period is parecoxib:

Table 3.8 Relative and absolute contraindications to the use of NSAIDs in anaesthesia

Relative contraindications	Absolute contraindications
• High risk of intraoperative bleeding e.g. vascular surgery	• Pre-existing renal dysfunction, hyperkalaemia
• Concurrent use of ACE inhibitors, anticoagulants, nephrotoxic drugs	• Cardiac failure
• Hepatic dysfunction	• Severe hepatic dysfunction
• Bleeding disorders	• History of GI bleeding
• Elderly (>65 years)	• Hypersensitivity to NSAIDs
• Pregnancy and during lactation	• Aspirin induced asthma
• Asthma	

- a selective COX-2 inhibitor, with predominantly analgesic activity, usually given IV, but can be given IM;
- initial IV dose 40 mg, subsequent doses 20–40 mg, 6–12 hourly, maximum 80 mg/day for 2 days – reduce dose by 50% in elderly;
- effective after orthopaedic surgery, has opioid-sparing effects after abdominal surgery;
- no effect on ventilation or cardiovascular function;
- not subject to the Misuse of Drugs Regulations.

Paracetamol

An analgesic and antipyretic with little anti-inflammatory action, but usually classified with NSAIDs. It inhibits prostaglandin synthesis, mainly in the CNS. It is well absorbed when taken orally with minimal adverse effect on the gastrointestinal tract. Widely used orally for the treatment of mild to moderate pain in a dose of 1 g 4–6 hourly, maximum 4 g/day and is often incorporated into compound preparations with aspirin or codeine. An intravenous preparation is available containing 10 mg/mL, in 100 mL vials (1 g). The dose is the same as for the oral preparation, can be infused over 15 min and is effective in 5–10 min. It is the safest of all analgesics but patients may need reassurance that regular dosing of 1 g every 6 hours is not associated with hepatic toxicity.

Table 3.9 Commonly used anti-emetic drugs, dose, and ideal timing

Type of drug	Example	Usual dose	Timing	Notes
Dopamine antagonists	Metoclopramide	10 mg orally or IV	End of surgery	Pro-kinetic, extrapyramidal side effects
5-hydroxytryptamine antagonists	Ondansetron	4–8 mg orally or IV	End of surgery	More effective at treating established vomiting
Antihistamines	Cyclizine	50 mg IM or IV	End of surgery	Cyclizine has anti-vagal properties, may cause a tachycardia. Painful when given IM
Anticholinergics	Hyoscine	1 mg transdermal patch	>4 h before surgery	
Corticosteroid	Dexamethasone	4–8 mg IV	At induction	Causes perineal burning sensation if given to awake patients

Anti-emetics

A significant proportion of patients experience postoperative nausea and vomiting (PONV), ranging from 25–80% in different patient groups. This has many adverse consequences including increased patient anxiety and dissatisfaction, increased pain, risk of aspiration, wound dehiscence, and potential delayed discharge after day-case surgery. However, it is not cost effective to give anti-emetic drugs to all patients and would potentially expose many patients to unwanted side effects. Whether the type of surgery influences the risk of PONV is still debated. It has been shown that there are four independent risk factors that can help to predict a patient's likelihood of experiencing PONV, and therefore which patients may benefit from prophylactic anti-emetics, or an altered anaesthetic technique. These are:

- female sex;
- being a non-smoker;
- previous history of PONV or motion sickness;
- opioids as part of the anaesthetic technique.

The incidence of PONV increases with the number of risk factors and is approximately 10%, 20%, 40%, 60%, and 80% in patients with zero, one, two, three or four risk factors respectively. A scoring system that allocates one point for each of the four risk factors listed above has been devised (the Apfel score) to try to stratify an individual patient's risk of PONV and guide prophylaxis. Patients who score:

- 0 or 1 points have a low risk of PONV and should not routinely receive anti-emetics;
- 2 or more points have a high risk of PONV and should receive combination therapy (use drugs with different modes of action).

For patients with two or more risk factors, consideration should also be given to altering the anaesthetic technique to one associated with a lower incidence of PONV, for example a regional anaesthetic technique, general anaesthesia with TIVA, avoiding opioids where possible. Even combination therapy is not certain to prevent PONV and patients may need further treatment as they recover from anaesthesia.

Some of the more commonly used anti-emetic drugs are detailed in Table 3.9.

Local anaesthetic drugs

When applied to nervous tissue these drugs cause a reversible loss of the ability to conduct nerve impulses. They can be given by a variety of routes, including topically, subcutaneously or directly adjacent to nerves.

Mechanism of action

At rest, a nerve cell has a transmembrane electrical potential (voltage) of -70 mV, and is said to be polarized. Noxious, mechanical, thermal, or chemical stimuli, depending on their intensity, cause sodium ions (Na^+) to enter the cell. If the stimulus is of sufficient intensity, a depolarization threshold is reached that triggers sodium channels to open allowing Na^+ to flood into the cell. As a result, the cell's membrane potential is reversed to $+20\,mV$ and an 'action potential' is initiated. This local change in the cell's membrane electrical potential causes adjacent voltage-gated sodium channels to open altering that segment's membrane potential, propagating the action potential along the nerve. The membrane is rapidly repolarized to the resting level by loss of potassium ions (K^+) from within the cell, followed by active pumping out of Na^+ in exchange for K^+ by the Na/K ATPase pump. During repolarization no action potential can be propagated by that section of nerve, thus ensuring unidirectional travel of action potentials. Not all stimuli are sufficient to reach the threshold, and so some will not lead to an action potential being initiated or propagated. Action potentials are 'all-or-nothing' events, and all of equal magnitude. Consequently, the strength of a nervous impulse is solely dependent on the frequency of action potentials.

In myelinated nerves the rate of conduction is vastly increased as the action potential 'jumps' between the nodes of Ranvier, a process known as 'saltatory conduction'.

Local anaesthetic drugs work by blocking the voltage-gated sodium channels from within the nerve cell, preventing entry of sodium and subsequent depolarization so that no action potentials can be initiated or propagated.

Local anaesthetic drugs exist in two forms: ionized and unionized. When a local anaesthetic is given, the majority will exist as the ionized form but, in order to cross the cell membrane, they have to be in the unionized form. This change occurs after injection because of a relatively higher pH in tissues (7.4 compared to 6.0 in solution). However, intracellular pH is lower (7.1) and so a greater proportion returns to its ionized form. It is this form that is attracted to, and then blocks, the sodium channels. Clearly, the degree of unionized drug will have an effect on the speed of onset. This can be further increased by using a higher concentration of the drug.

The duration of action will be determined by what proportion is protein bound, generally the greater the binding to membrane proteins, the longer the duration of action. Local blood supply will also have an effect as this will affect the speed of removal of the drug. The degree of lipid solubility will determine potency by influencing the membrane penetration by the drug but will also result in a tendency for greater toxicity.

Following the injection of a local anaesthetic drug, there is always a predictable sequence to the onset of effects as small diameter nerves are blocked before large diameter ones, and unmyelinated nerves are blocked before myelinated ones. Consequently when a regional anaesthetic technique is used, the order of onset of the block is:

- autonomic fibres – vasodilatation;
- temperature;
- pain;
- touch;
- motor – paralysis.

This accounts for the warm feeling that patients frequently notice at the onset of spinal or epidural anaesthesia, and that under some circumstances patients feel no pain but can still move their legs.

Individual drugs

Local anaesthetic drugs can be divided into two groups on the basis of their chemical structure:

- esters: amethocaine, benzocaine, cocaine;
- amides: lignocaine, bupivacaine, prilocaine.

The esters were the first drugs to be introduced into clinical practice. They are relatively more toxic, allergenic, and unstable than their modern counterparts the amides. Their main use today is to provide topical anaesthesia.

Amethocaine

Available as a 4% gel (Ametop) that is applied topically at the site of intended intravenous cannulation, and is effective in 45 min. More dilute solutions are available to provide topical anaesthesia of the conjunctiva.

Cocaine

Available as a paste and spray, in concentrations of 4–10%, and mainly used to provide topical anaesthesia of the nasal cavity. It has sympathomimetic properties, which are advantageous, for example profound vasoconstriction reduces bleeding and prolongs its action, but is also responsible for its toxicity and risk of arrhythmias.

Lidocaine

A commonly used local anaesthetic in a variety of techniques including topically, by infiltration, nerve blocks, epidural and spinal anaesthesia. Consequently it is available in a range of concentrations, 0.5–10%, to suit all situations. It is often combined with adrenaline (see below). It has a relatively fast onset and medium duration of effect. The currently accepted maximum safe dose is:

- 3 mg/kg, maximum 200 mg (without adrenaline);
- 6–7 mg/kg, maximum 500 mg (with adrenaline).

These doses should be reduced if the patient is elderly, frail or shocked. It can also be used in the treatment of VF/VT refractory to defibrillation (100 mg IV) when amiodarone is unavailable. As with all amide local anaesthetics it is metabolized in the liver.

Bupivacaine

Bupivacaine has a slower onset but a longer duration of action than lignocaine, and is widely used for nerve blocks, epidural and spinal anaesthesia, particularly in obstetric anaesthesia. It is available as either 0.25% or 0.5% solutions, with or without adrenaline, as a hyperbaric 0.5% preservative free solution with 8% dextrose for use in spinal anaesthesia, and as 0.1% and 0.125% solutions, which are used for epidural infusion to provide pain relief during labour and postoperatively. The current maximum safe dose is 2 mg/kg, with or without adrenaline, in any 4 hour period. Bupivacaine is significantly more cardiotoxic than other amide local anaesthetics and toxicity is difficult to treat (see Chapter 5 for the management of local anaesthetic toxicity).

Bupivacaine molecules can exist in two forms that are "mirror images" of each other, termed stereoisomers. The two different forms of the molecule are described according to various conventions, the most commonly used being based upon their ability to rotate polarized light, either; + or d (dextrorotatory), – or l (laevorotatory). Bupivacaine is produced for clinical use as a racemic mixture, meaning it contains both isomers in equal quantities, levo-bupivacaine (chirocaine®) is the pure L isomer. Whichever form is used, the doses are the same, but levo-bupivacaine has the advantage of significantly reduced cardiotoxicity.

Ropivacaine

An amide local anaesthetic which, like bupivacaine, can exist as two stereoisomers. It is prepared as a single isomer and has the same potency and duration of action as bupivacaine, but lower toxicity. It also has the advantage of reduced duration and intensity of motor block, which makes it useful for postoperative analgesia.

Prilocaine

Closely related to lidocaine, its advantages are rapid onset and reduced toxicity for a given dose. It is a component of EMLA, a *e*utectic *m*ixture of *l*ocal *a*naesthetics. This is a cream that contains lidocaine and prilocaine in equal proportions (25 mg of each per gram). It is applied to the skin and produces surface analgesia in approximately 60 min. In this form it is used to reduce the pain associated with venepuncture, particularly in children. A 2% solution of hyperbaric prilocaine has recently been introduced for spinal anaesthesia for short procedures. (A gel containing 4% amethocaine is also available for surface analgesia.)

A synopsis of the drugs used for local and regional anaesthesia is given in Table 3.10.

Adrenaline (epinephrine)

Adrenaline is a potent vasoconstrictor as a result of its action at α-adrenergic receptors and is added to local anaesthetics to reduce blood flow at the site of injection. This has several beneficial effects, notably to reduce the rate of absorption, reduce toxicity and extend the duration of action. This is most effective during infiltration anaesthesia and nerve blocks, and less effective in epidurals or spinals. Some authorities recommend that solutions containing adrenaline should never be used intrathecally. Only very small concentrations of adrenaline are required to obtain intense vasoconstriction. The concentration is expressed as the weight of adrenaline (g) per volume of solution (mL). Concentrations commonly used with local anaesthetics range from 1:80 000 to 1:200 000.

Local anaesthetics containing vasoconstrictors should not be used around extremities (for example, fingers, toes, penis) because of the risk of vasoconstriction causing tissue necrosis.

The maximum safe dose of adrenaline in an adult is 250 μg – that is, 20 mL of 1:80 000 or 50 mL of 1:200 000. This should be reduced by 50% in patients with ischaemic heart disease.

Table 3.10 Local anaesthetic drugs

Drug	Dose	Speed of onset	Duration of action	Comments
Lidocaine	Plain: 3 mg/kg, max 200 mg With adrenaline: 6 mg/kg, max 500 mg	Rapid	60–180 min, depending on the technique used	Used: topically, infiltration, nerve blocks, IVRA, epidurally, intrathecally
Bupivacaine	± adrenaline: 2 mg/kg, max 150 mg in any 4 h period	Nerve block: up to 40 min Epidurally: 15–20 min Intrathecal: 30 s	Up to 24 h 3–4 h, dose dependent 2–3 h, dose dependent	Mainly used for nerve blocks, epidurally and intrathecally Relatively cardiotoxic
Levo-bupivacaine	An isomer of bupivacaine; most properties very similar, but less cardiotoxic.			This allows slightly higher doses to be given
Ropivacaine	3 mg/kg, max 200 mg	Similar to bupivacaine	For the same concentration and technique, shorter than bupivacaine	At lower concentrations, relatively less intense motor block than bupivacaine

IVRA: intravenous regional anaesthesia.

Calculation of doses

For any drug it is essential that the correct dose is given and that the maximum safe dose is never exceeded. This can be confusing with local anaesthetic drugs as the volume containing the required dose will vary depending upon the concentration (expressed in per cent) and a range of concentrations exists for each drug. The relationship between concentration, volume and dose is given by the formula:

$$\text{Concentration (\%)} \times \text{Volume (ml)} \times 10 = \text{dose (mg)}$$

Intravenous fluids

During anaesthesia fluids are given intravenously to replace losses due to surgery, and to provide the patient's normal daily requirements. Three types are used: crystalloids, colloids and blood and its components.

Crystalloids

These are solutions of crystalline solids in water. The solutions can be considered in two groups; those that contain electrolytes in a similar composition to plasma, have an osmolality similar to plasma and are often referred to as being isotonic, and those that contain less or no electrolytes (hypotonic) but contain glucose to ensure that they have an osmolality similar to plasma. A summary of the composition of the most commonly used is shown in Table 3.11. Once these fluids are given they are redistributed amongst the various body fluid compartments, the extent depending on their composition. For example, 0.9% saline is distributed throughout the intravascular and interstitial volumes (extracellular fluid compartment, ECF) in proportion to their size. After 15–30 min, only 25–30% of the volume administered remains intravascular. Therefore, if such a fluid is used to restore the circulating volume, three to four times the deficit will need to be given. If a hypotonic solution is given, for example 5% glucose, once the glucose is metabolized the remaining fluid is distributed throughout the entire body water (extracellular and intracellular

Table 3.11 **Composition of crystalloids**

Crystalloid	Na$^+$ (mmol/L)	K$^+$ (mmol/L)	Ca^{++} (mmol/L)	Cl$^-$ (mmol/L)	HCO$_3^-$ (mmol/L)	pH	Osmolality (mosmol/L)
Hartmann's	131	5	4	112	29*	6.5	281
0.9% sodium chloride	154	0	0	154	0	5.5	300
4% glucose plus 0.18% sodium chloride	31	0	0	31	0	4.5	284
5% glucose	0	0	0	0	0	4.1	278

*Present as lactate which is metabolized to bicarbonate by the liver.

volumes) and less than 10% will remain intravascular. Glucose-containing solutions are a way of treating dehydration as a result of water losses but may cause hyponatraemia. They are not routinely used perioperatively. Traditionally, 0.9% saline solution has been widely used in the perioperative period and as the first line for emergency fluid resuscitation. However large volumes cause hyperchloraemic metabolic acidosis, as although regarded as isotonic, it contains a greater concentration of chloride than plasma.

Recently, consensus guidelines on IV fluid therapy for adult surgical patients (GIFTASUP) have been issued. These recommend:

- When crystalloid resuscitation or replacement is indicated, balanced salt solutions, for example Ringer's lactate/acetate or Hartmann's solution, should replace 0.9% saline to reduce the risk of hyperchloraemic acidosis.
- To meet maintenance requirements, adult patients should receive sodium 50–100 mmol/day, potassium 40–80 mmol/day in 1.5–2.5 L of water by the oral, enteral or parenteral route (or a combination of routes). Additional amounts should only be given to correct deficit or continuing losses.
- Excessive losses from gastric aspiration/vomiting should be treated with an appropriate crystalloid solution, which includes an appropriate potassium supplement. Hypochloraemia is an indication for the use of 0.9% saline, with sufficient additions of potassium and care must be taken not to produce sodium overload. Losses from diarrhoea/ileostomy/small bowel fistula/ileus/obstruction should be replaced volume for volume with Hartmann's or Ringer-Lactate/

acetate type solutions. 'Saline depletion', for example due to excessive diuretic exposure, is best managed with a balanced electrolyte solution such as Hartmann's. For further details see useful information section.

Saline is also available as a hypertonic solution consisting of between 1.8% and 7.5% sodium chloride solutions. When given, these raise the osmolality of the ECF (mainly the intravascular component) and create a gradient such that water moves from the intracellular fluid (ICF) into the plasma. The intravascular volume is expanded by a greater volume than the volume of hypertonic solution given, for example 250 mL 7.5% saline results in plasma expansion by up to 1.5 L. If given repeatedly they will result in intracellular dehydration, which must be corrected subsequently. There is no evidence for their routine use during in the perioperative period, however, they may have a role in resuscitating patients with traumatic brain injury, where they appear to reduce cerebral oedema, restore cerebral perfusion and help reduce neuronal injury.

Colloids

These are suspensions of high molecular weight particles. The most commonly used are derived from gelatin (for example, Haemaccel®, Gelofusine®), protein (albumin) or hydroxyethyl starch, HES (for example, hetastarch, Voluven®). Colloids primarily expand the intravascular volume and can initially be given in a volume similar to the estimated deficit to maintain the circulating volume. However, they have a finite life in the plasma and will eventually either be metabolized or excreted,

Table 3.12 Composition of colloids

Colloid	Average molecular weight (kDa)	Na$^+$ (mmol/L)	K$^+$ (mmol/L)	Ca^{++} (mmol/L)	Cl$^-$ (mmol/L)	HCO$_3^-$ (mmol/L)	pH	Osmolality (mosmol/L)
Haemaccel	35	145	5	6.2	145	0	7.3	350
Gelofusine	35	154	0.4	0.4	125	0	7.4	465
Albumin	69	130–160	2	0	120	0	6.7–7.3	270–300
Hetastarch	450	154	0	0	154	0	5.5	310
Voluven	130	154	0	0	154	0	4.0–5.5	308
Volulyte	130	137	4	1.5*	110	34**	5.7–6.5	286

*Calcium replaced with magnesium, ** bicarbonate replaced with acetate.

and therefore need replacing. A summary of their composition is shown in Table 3.12. There is no limit on the volume of gelatins that can be given (provided that haemoglobin concentration is maintained!), however, of the colloids, they have the greatest tendency to release histamine and may rarely cause anaphylaxis (1–2 cases per 10 000 units given). Hydroxyethyl starch products differ widely, particularly in terms of their molecular weight (70–650 kDa) and resistance to breakdown (expressed as their degree of substitution (DS) of glucose for hydroxyethyl units), which in turn affects their duration in the plasma. Current products have a MW of 130–200 kDa and DS of 0.4. This has reduced the early problems of renal failure, coagulopathy and bleeding, but HES is still associated with reductions in factor VIII. Itching may also be a problem in some patients and may be prolonged. The volume of starches that can be given is limited to 30–50 mL/kg, depending on the formulation used. A preparation combining HES with hypertonic (7.2%) saline is also available (HyperHAES®).

Blood and blood components

Before use, donated whole blood is generally processed into the following products to allow the most appropriate components to be given:

- *Red cells in optimal additive solution (SAG-M).* A red cell concentrate to which a mixture of saline, adenine and glucose and mannitol has been added. This improves both red cell survival and flow characteristics. Each unit contains approximately 300 mL with a haematocrit of 50–70% and will raise a patient's Hb by roughly 1 g/dL. White cells are routinely removed in the UK to prevent the risk of prion disease transmission.
- *Platelet concentrates.* Supplied either as 'units' containing 50–60 mL (55×10^9 platelets) or as bags equivalent to four units. Four units or one bag will raise the platelet count by $30–40 \times 10^9$/L. It is given via a standard giving set *without* the use of a microaggregate filter, as this will result in the loss of significant numbers of platelets.
- *Fresh frozen plasma (FFP).* One unit consists of the plasma separated from a single donation, usually 200–250 mL, and frozen within 6 hours. It contains normal levels of clotting factors (except factor VIII, 70% normal). An adult dose is 4 units. It should be infused as soon as it has thawed.
- *Cryoprecipitate.* On controlled thawing of FFP a precipitate is formed, which is collected and suspended in plasma. It contains large amounts of factor VIII and fibrinogen. It is supplied as a pooled donation from six packs of FFP in one unit and must be used as soon as possible after thawing.

Risks of blood and blood-product transfusions

All blood donations are routinely tested for hepatitis B surface antigen, hepatitis C, syphilis, HTLV, and antibodies to HIV. However, a period exists between exposure to viruses and the development of antibodies. The resultant infected red cells would not be detected by current screening techniques. The risk is very small, and has been estimated for hepatitis B at $1:10^5$ and for HIV at $1:10^6$ units transfused.

In order to try to eliminate these risks, techniques now exist for using the patient's own blood in the perioperative period. This also has the advantage of reducing the chances of, but not eliminating, the wrong unit of blood being transfused.

- *Predepositing blood.* Over a period of 4 weeks prior to surgery, the patient builds up a bank of 2–4 units of blood for retransfusion perioperatively.
- *Preoperative haemodilution.* Following induction of anaesthesia 0.5–1.5 L of blood is removed and replaced with colloid. This can then be transfused at the end of surgery.
- *Cell savers.* These devices collect blood lost during surgery via a suction system; the red cells are separated, washed and resuspended, ready for retransfusion to the patient (see Chapter 2).

📖 FURTHER USEFUL INFORMATION

British Medical Association and the Royal Pharmaceutical Society of Great Britain. *British National Formulary (BNF).* London: British Medical Association and the Royal Pharmaceutical Society of Great Britain. (Current issue available at BNF website: www.bnf.org/.)

Peck TE, Hill SA, Williams M (eds). *Pharmacology for anaesthesia and intensive care,* 3rd edn. New York: Cambridge University Press, 2008

www.aagbi.org/
[The Association of Anaesthetists of Great Britain and Ireland.]

www.aagbi.org/publications/guidelines/docs/bloodtransfusion06.pdf
[Association of Anaesthetists guidelines on blood transfusion and component therapy, 2005.]

www.carg.cochrane.org/en/index.html
[This site contains systematic reviews of aspects of anaesthetic practice.]

www.frca.co.uk/
[AnaesthesiaUK. The most popular website for trainees in anaesthesia].

www.mhra.gov.uk/
[Medicines and Healthcare Products Regulatory Agency. This agency ensures that medicines, healthcare products and medical equipment meet appropriate standards of safety, quality, performance and effectiveness, and are used safely. Site contains latest drug and device hazards.]

www.rcoa.ac.uk/
[The Royal College of Anaesthetists. These first two sites are a must if you want to have the latest national UK guidance on anaesthetic practice.]

www.renal.org/pages/media/download_gallery/GIFTASUP%20FINAL_05_01_09.pdf
[The full British Consensus Guidelines on Intravenous Fluid Therapy for Adult Surgical Patients.]

www.shotuk.org/
[Serious Hazards of Transfusion (SHOT). Contains latest UK data.]

All websites last accessed February 2012.

? SELF-ASSESSMENT

Short-answer questions

3.1 Describe the sequence of pharmacological and clinical events when a dose of suxamethonium is given? What are the important side effects?

3.2 How do non-steroidal anti-inflammatory drugs work? What are the relative and absolute contraindications to their use?

3.3 What factors increase the risk of postoperative nausea and vomiting (PONV)? How can these be used to stratify an individual patient's risk of PONV and guide prophylaxis? Describe the drugs and doses that can be used to treat PONV.

3.4 Describe the central effects of opioid drugs. How can these be reversed?

3.5 Describe how a nerve impulse is transmitted. How do local anaesthetic drugs affect this? How much lidocaine is contained in 15 ml of a 0.75% solution? What is the maximum safe dose, with and without adrenaline?

True/false questions

3.1 When using an IV drug to induce anaesthesia:
   a propofol causes hypotension and respiratory depression;
   b propofol is cumulative after repeated doses;
   c thiopentone causes involuntary movement and hiccoughs;
   d ketamine is antanalgesic.

3.2 Suxamethonium:
   a is a non-depolarizing neuromuscular blocking drug;
   b has a rapid onset and short duration of action;
   c can be reversed with neostigmine;
   d may cause hypokalaemia.

3.3 With respect to local anaesthetic drugs:
   a they are only active in the unionized form;
   b when used for regional anaesthesia, sensory block precedes motor block;
   c lidocaine is less toxic than bupivacaine;
   d the maximum safe dose of lidocaine is 6 to 7 mg/kg.

3.4 Morphine:
   a is more effective against visceral pain than pain after trauma;
   b when given IV has a peak effect in < 5 min;
   c is a Schedule 3 drug;
   d causes pupillary dilatation.

3.5 When using inhalational anaesthesia:
   a an adequate depth of anaesthesia for surgery can be achieved reliably using nitrous oxide alone;
   b the minimum alveolar concentration (MAC) is a measure of anaesthetic potency;
   c speed of onset is faster with drugs that are more soluble in the blood;
   d the most suitable drug for an inhalational induction of anaesthesia is isoflurane.

4

The practice of general anaesthesia

There should be a smooth, controlled sequence of preplanned events from the time patients arrive in the anaesthetic room until they leave. This chapter aims to outline how, by applying the knowledge and skills from the previous chapters, the anaesthetist achieves this, thereby minimizing the risks of both anaesthesia and surgery. The descriptions given follow as closely as possible the sequence of events as they might be expected to occur during a normal anaesthetic.

Preoperative checks

Checking the anaesthetic machine

It is the responsibility of every anaesthetist to check that the anaesthetic machine, monitors, breathing system and any ancillary equipment will function in the manner expected at the beginning of each operating session. The main danger is that the anaesthetic machine appears to perform normally but in fact is delivering a hypoxic mixture to the patient. Most modern integrated anaesthesia machines perform a 'self-test' when first switched on and do not need to be retested by the user. A check of the gas supply, patency and lack of gas leaks in the breathing system is essential. The function, calibration and alarm settings on the monitors should also be checked. The AAGBI publish a document entitled *Checking Anaesthetic Equipment* that gives more comprehensive details. A record should be kept of each check of the anaesthetic machine and equipment. Appropriate procedures must also be in place to deal safely with any machine failure.

Checking the patient

Anaesthesia and surgery are not without risk. The World Health Organisation (WHO) has reported that in the industrialized countries,

Clinical Anaesthesia Lecture Notes, Fourth Edition. Carl Gwinnutt and Matthew Gwinnutt.
© 2012 John Wiley & Sons, Ltd. Published 2012 by John Wiley & Sons, Ltd.

major complications occur in 3–16% of inpatient surgical procedures and permanent disability or death in 0.4–0.8%. To try and reduce this degree of harm, the 'Safe Surgery Saves Lives' project was introduced. One of the key components of this is the use of a 'Surgical Safety Checklist', which is completed in three stages:

- before the induction of anaesthesia ('sign in');
- before the start of the surgical intervention (skin incision or equivalent) ('time out');
- before the team leaves the operating theatre (or at skin closure or its equivalent) ('sign out').

Sign in

1 When the patient arrives in the anaesthetic room, the anaesthetist and the anaesthetist's assistant must confirm the patient's identity, usually with the patient, the patient's wrist band and case notes. The nature of the planned operation, site, and side (if appropriate) is confirmed with the patient and a check is made to ensure the correct surgical site is clearly marked. The consent form is checked to ensure the correct details are entered and it is signed appropriately by the patient and surgical team. This is usually done verbally but occasionally an unconscious patient may need surgery, for example an intensive care patient. Great care should be taken and the above checks performed preferably by both the anaesthetist and surgeon.
2 A record is made that the anaesthetic machine has been checked along with the drugs required for the case.
3 A specific check is made of any known allergies the patient may have.
4 A specific check is made to ensure that any problems with airway management have been identified.
5 Anticipated blood loss and availability of blood is checked.

Preparation for anaesthesia

Several things now happen, often simultaneously:

- monitoring equipment is attached to the patient;
- IV access is obtained;
- the patient is preoxygenated.

Once all of these have been achieved satisfactorily, the patient is anaesthetised.

Monitoring the patient

This should commence before the induction of anaesthesia and continue until the patient has recovered from the effects of anaesthesia, and the information generated should be recorded in the patient's notes. The type and number of monitors used depend upon a variety of factors including:

- type of operation and operative technique;
- anaesthetic technique used;
- present and previous health of the patient;
- equipment available and the anaesthetist's ability to use it;
- preferences of the anaesthetist;
- any research being undertaken.

The AAGBI recommends certain monitoring devices as *essential* for the safe conduct of anaesthesia. These are ECG, non-invasive blood pressure (NIBP), pulse oximeter, capnography, and vapour concentration analysis. Clearly the latter two are only used after general anaesthesia has commenced. In addition, a peripheral nerve stimulator should be *immediately available*. Finally, additional equipment *will be required* in certain cases, to monitor, for example invasive blood pressure, urine output, CVP, and various haemodynamic parameters.

Recent recommendations from NICE are that all patients should have their temperature measured before induction of anaesthesia, and surgery should not be started (unless there is a critical need) if it is below 36 °C. Subsequently the patient's temperature should be measured every 30 min. Active warming should be used as described below.

There is good evidence that monitoring reduces the risks of adverse incidents and accidents. The combination of pulse oximetry, capnography, and blood pressure monitoring will detect the majority of serious incidents before there has been serious harm to the patient. Ultimately, monitoring supplements clinical observation; there is no substitute for the presence of a trained and experienced anaesthetist throughout the entire operative procedure.

Monitoring is not without its own potential hazards:

- faulty equipment may endanger the patient, for example from electrocution secondary to faulty earthing;

- the anaesthetist may act on faulty data, instituting inappropriate treatment;
- the patient may be harmed by the complications of the technique to establish invasive monitoring, for example pneumothorax following central venous catheterization.

Ultimately, too many monitors may distract the anaesthetist from recognizing problems occurring in other areas.

Intravenous access

The superficial veins on the back of the hand (*dorsal metacarpal veins*) and forearm (*cephalic and basilic veins*) are most commonly used for IV access. Veins in the antecubital fossa tend to be used either in an emergency situation or when attempts to cannulate peripheral veins have failed. It must be remembered that the brachial artery, the median nerve, and branches of the medial and lateral cutaneous nerves of the arm are in close proximity to the antecubital veins and easily damaged by needles or extravasated drugs. A cannula must not be sited in a patient's arm on the side where the patient has undergone clearance of axillary lymph nodes for malignant disease unless there is no alternative because of the risk of exacerbating lymphoedema. The size of cannula inserted will depend upon its purpose: large-diameter cannulas are required for giving fluid rapidly; smaller ones are adequate for giving drugs and maintenance fluids. Peripheral venous cannulation is an essential skill, best learnt under the supervision of an anaesthetist, rather than reading about it! Complications of peripheral venous cannulation are shown in Table 4.1.

A small amount of local anaesthetic (0.2 mL lignocaine 1%) should be infiltrated into the skin at the site chosen for venepuncture using a 25 g (0.5 mm) needle, particularly if a large (>18 g, 1.2 mm) cannula is used. This reduces pain and makes the patient less likely to move and less resistant to further attempts.

As with any procedure where there is a risk of contact with body fluids, gloves must be worn by the operator.

Central venous cannulation

This usually takes place after the patient has been anaesthetised to allow monitoring of the cardiovascular system or to give certain drugs (for example, inotropes). Rarely, it is required before the anaesthetic is given because of lack of or inadequate peripheral venous access (for example in a patient who has a history of IV drug abuse). It is included at this point for completeness. There are many different types of equipment and approaches to the central veins, and the following is intended as an outline. It is now recommended that an ultrasound scanner is used to detect central veins and guide the insertion of the needle into the vein (Fig. 4.1).

The internal jugular vein

This approach is associated with the highest incidence of success (95%), and a low rate of complications (Table 4.2). The right internal jugular offers certain advantages: there is a 'straight line' to the heart, the apical pleura does not rise as high on this side, and the main thoracic duct is on the left.

Table 4.1 Complications of peripheral venous cannulation

- *Failure:* attempt cannulation distally in a limb and work proximally. If multiple attempts are required, fluid or drugs will not leak from previous puncture sites.
- *Haematoma:* usually secondary to the above with inadequate pressure applied over the puncture site to prevent bleeding, and made worse by forgetting to remove the tourniquet!
- *Extravasation of fluid or drugs:* failing to recognize that the cannula is not within the vein before use. May cause damage to the surrounding tissues.
- *Damage to local structures:* secondary to poor technique and lack of knowledge of the local anatomy.
- *Air embolus:* most likely following cannulation of a central vein (see below).
- *Shearing of the cannula:* usually a result of trying to reintroduce the needle after it has been withdrawn. The safest action is to withdraw the whole cannula and attempt again at another site.
- *Thrombophlebitis:* related to the length of time the vein is in use and irritation caused by the substances flowing through it. High concentrations of drugs and fluids with extremes of pH or high osmolality are the main causes, e.g. antibiotics, calcium chloride, sodium bicarbonate. Once a vein shows signs of thrombophlebitis (i.e. tender, red and deteriorating flow) the cannula must be removed to prevent subsequent infection or thrombosis.

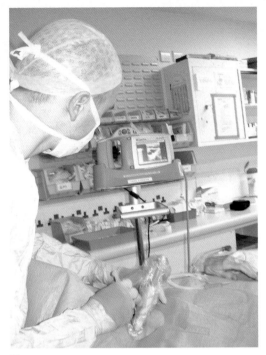

(a)

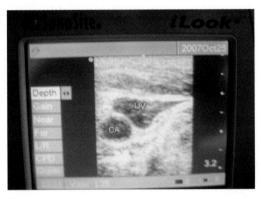

(b)

Figure 4.1 (a) CVP catheter being inserted using ultrasound guidance. (b) Ultrasound screen showing relative positions of the internal jugular vein (IJV) and carotid artery (CA).

Subclavian vein

This can be approached by both the supra- and infraclavicular routes. Both are technically more difficult than the internal jugular route and there is a significant incidence of causing a pneumothorax (approximately 2%). The main advantages of this route are comfort for the patient and low risk of infection during long-term use.

Table 4.2 **Complications of internal jugular vein cannulation**

- arterial puncture and bleeding causing haematoma or haemothorax
- air embolus
- venous thrombosis
- pneumothorax
- thoracic duct injury (left side) and chylothorax
- hydrothorax if the catheter is intrapleural and fluid given
- bacteraemia
- septicaemia
- soft tissue infection at puncture site
- injury to nerves:
  o brachial plexus
  o recurrent laryngeal
  o phrenic

Bilateral attempts at central venous cannulation must not be made because of the risk of airway obstruction due to haematoma formation in the neck or bilateral pneumothoraces.

Equipment for central venous catheterization

The techniques commonly used for percutaneous cannulation of the central veins are:

- *Catheter over needle.* Similar to a peripheral IV cannula, the main difference is that it is longer so that it reaches from the site of insertion to the superior vena cava.
- *Seldinger technique.* The vein is punctured initially percutaneously using a small-diameter needle. A flexible guidewire is then passed through the needle into the vein and the needle carefully withdrawn, leaving the wire behind. The catheter is now passed over the wire into the vein, sometimes preceded by a dilator. The advantage of this method is that the initial use of a small needle increases the chance of successful venepuncture and reduces the risk of damage to the vein.

Whenever a central venous catheter is inserted, a chest X-ray must be taken to ensure that the catheter is correctly positioned with the tip at the junction of the superior vena cava and right atrium and that a pneumothorax has not been caused.

Arterial cannulation

This can be performed under local anaesthesia before the patient is anaesthetised or once the patient has been anaesthetised. The radial artery is most commonly used (femoral and brachial are also used) as it is superficial, compressible and there is usually good collateral circulation to the hand via the ulnar artery. It has been advocated that Allen's test to check the adequacy of the ulnar circulation is performed before radial artery cannulation.

Technique of cannulation

The wrist is fully supinated and dorsiflexed about 60°, often over a small support. The skin is cleansed appropriately and the position of the radial artery identified by palpation at the level of the proximal wrist skin crease. If local anaesthetic is used, a small volume (0.2 ml) is injected using a 25 g needle over and to either side of the artery. Two techniques are used to cannulate the artery:

- Direct puncture using a catheter over needle, either a non-ported IV cannula or a specifically designed arterial cannula with a built-in on/off switch. The skin is punctured at an angle of 20–30° and the needle point advanced toward as the artery. As the artery is punctured, arterial blood fills the flashback chamber. The needle should then be lowered to about 10° and advanced a further 1–2 mm to ensure the tip of the cannula lies within the artery. The cannula is then advanced off the needle into the artery.
- Seldinger technique. The artery is punctured directly with the needle as described above. Successful puncture is confirmed by getting pulsatile blood from the hub of the needle. The guidewire is advanced through the needle and the needle carefully withdrawn, leaving the wire behind. The catheter is now passed over the wire into the artery.

Once the cannula is in place, it is usually sutured to reduce the risk of accidental removal and covered with a transparent, sterile dressing.

Complications of arterial cannulation include bleeding, infection, thrombosis and aneurysm formation.

Preoxygenation

At the end of expiration, the lungs contain a significant volume of air that acts as a reservoir (the functional residual capacity, FRC). Amongst other things, this prevents hypoxaemia during brief periods of breath-holding. However, breathing room air the vast majority of the FRC is nitrogen. The purpose of preoxygenation is to replace the nitrogen with oxygen, thereby significantly increasing the length of time a patient can be apnoeic (or not ventilated), without becoming hypoxic; effectively 'buying time' for both the patient and anaesthetist in case of difficulty. Preoxygenation is usually achieved by getting the patient to breathe 100% oxygen via a close-fitting facemask for about 3 minutes or until the oxygen concentration in expired gas exceeds 85%. In an emergency situation a reasonable degree of preoxygenation can be achieved by asking a cooperative patient to take four vital capacity breaths of 100% oxygen via an anaesthetic circuit with a tight-sealing facemask.

Induction of anaesthesia

Intravenous drugs are the most frequently used method of inducing anaesthesia. The drug dose is calculated, taking into account the patient's age and any comorbidities, and then given over 20–30 s. This method is generally preferred by both the patient, as consciousness is lost rapidly, and by the anaesthetist because pharyngeal reflexes are depressed allowing the insertion of an airway device. There are a number of potential disadvantages:

- Patients often become apnoeic. This may necessitate manual ventilation until spontaneous ventilation resumes.
- There will be a varying degree of hypotension. This will depend on the drug, dose used, speed given, and 'fitness' of the patient.
- There may be loss of airway patency. This can usually be overcome by a combination of basic airway opening manoeuvres, insertion of an oropharyngeal airway or supraglottic airway device.

Inhalational induction of anaesthesia is an alternative. It is achieved by the patient breathing a gradually increasing concentration of an inhalational drug in oxygen or a mixture of oxygen and nitrous oxide. Its advantages are that it can be used in:

- Patients with a lack of suitable veins. Rather than subject the patient to repeated attempts at venepuncture, anaesthesia is induced and, as most drugs are vasodilators, venepuncture is then possible.

- An uncooperative child, or patients with a needle phobia. Venous access can be obtained after induction.
- Patients with airway compromise, in which an IV drug may cause apnoea and loss of airway patency. Ventilation and oxygenation become impossible, with catastrophic results. Inhalation induction preserves spontaneous ventilation and if airway patency is threatened, further uptake of anaesthetic is prevented, limiting the problem.

Potential disadvantages include:

- Unconsciousness occurs more slowly than with an IV drug.
- Most inhalational drugs are unpleasant to breathe. Currently, sevoflurane is the most popular anaesthetic used for this technique.
- Hypotension and a fall in cardiac output occur with increasing concentrations. This may be difficult to treat until IV access is obtained.
- The combination of hypercapnia, as a result of respiratory depression and the vasodilator effect of these drugs lead to increased cerebral blood flow, making this technique unsuitable in patients with raised intracranial pressure.

As the concentration of inhalational drug increases, there is progressive reduction in the ventilatory activity of the intercostal muscles, muscle tone generally is also reduced and laryngeal reflexes are lost. The pupils start by becoming dilated, then slightly constricted and finally gradually dilate. This point is referred to as 'surgical anaesthesia'. Any further increase in depth of anaesthesia will result in diaphragmatic paralysis and cardiovascular collapse.

As well as the above, the anaesthetic will have effects on all of the other body systems, which will need appropriate monitoring.

Maintaining the airway

General anaesthesia frequently causes the patient's airway to become obstructed following loss of tone in the muscles of the tongue and pharynx (Fig. 4.2). The easiest way to restore patency is through basic airway manoeuvres; a

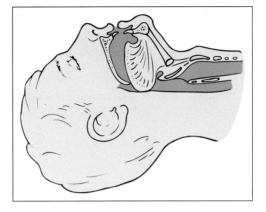

Figure 4.2 Sagittal section of the head and neck showing how the tongue contributes to airway obstruction.

combination of the head tilt, chin lift (Fig. 4.3) and jaw thrust (Fig. 4.4), in conjunction with an oro- or naso- pharyngeal airway. Although a patent airway can be maintained in the majority of patients in this manner it is increasingly uncommon as it severely restricts any further activity by the anaesthetist. This problem has been overcome by the use of a supraglottic airway device. The best method of providing and securing a clear airway in patients is tracheal intubation, but this is not appropriate in all patients.

Oropharyngeal airway

Estimate the size required by comparing the airway length with the vertical distance between the patient's incisor teeth (or if edentulous, the

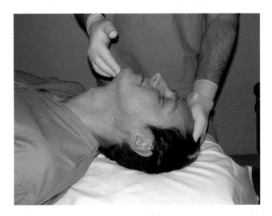

Figure 4.3 Head tilt, chin lift.

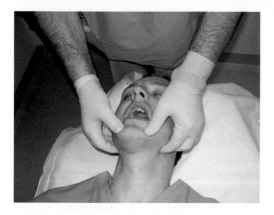

Figure 4.4 Jaw thrust. The application of pressure is behind the angles of the mandible. The thumbs can be used to open the mouth.

front of the mouth) and the angle of the jaw. Then insert, the airway initially 'upside down', as far as the back of the hard palate before rotating it 180° and fully inserting until the flange lies in front of the teeth, (or gums in an edentulous patient) (Fig. 4.5a–d).

Nasopharyngeal airway

Choose an appropriately sized airway, 7 mm for women, 8 mm for men, check the patency of the nostril to be used (usually the right) and lubricate the airway. The airway is then inserted along the floor of the nose, with the bevel facing medially to avoid catching the turbinates (Fig. 4.6a–c). A safety pin may be inserted through the flange to prevent inhalation of the airway. If obstruction is encountered, do not use force as severe bleeding may be provoked. Instead, try the other nostril.

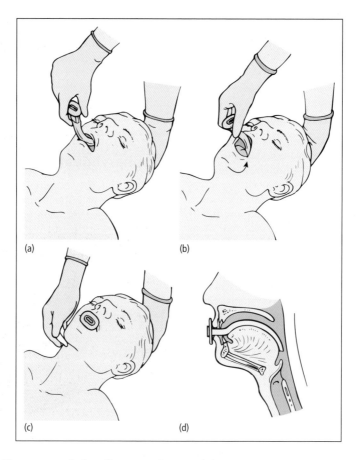

(a)

(b)

(c)

(d)

Figure 4.5 (a–d) The sequence for inserting an oropharyngeal airway.

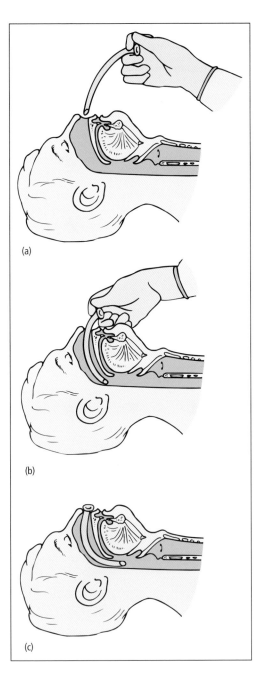

(a)

(b)

(c)

Figure 4.6 (a–c) The sequence for inserting a nasopharyngeal airway.

Problems with airways

- Although the techniques described so far will create and maintain a patent airway, they offer

no protection against aspiration of regurgitated gastric contents.
- Failure to maintain a patent airway: snoring, indrawing of the supraclavicular, suprasternal and intercostal spaces, use of the accessory muscles, or paradoxical respiratory movement (see-saw respiration) suggest obstruction.
- Inability to maintain a good seal between the patient's face and the mask, particularly in those without teeth.
- Fatigue, when holding the mask for prolonged periods.
- The anaesthetist not being free to deal with any other problems that may arise.

A supraglottic airway or tracheal intubation may be used to overcome these problems.

Facemasks

A facemask is used to ensure that the anaesthetic gas mixture is delivered to the patient. Leakage of gases is minimized by using one that provides a good seal. When holding a facemask in position with the index finger and thumb, the jaw thrust is achieved by lifting the angle of the mandible with the remaining fingers of one or both hands. The overall desired effect is that the patient's mandible is 'lifted' into the mask, rather than the mask being pushed into the face (Fig. 4.7). The patient can now breathe spontaneously or be ventilated.

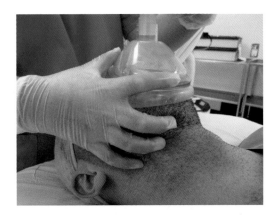

Figure 4.7 Mask being held on patient's face. Note the use of the little finger to apply a jaw thrust.

Supraglottic airway devices

These are widely used in spontaneously breathing patients as they overcome some of the problems associated with the techniques described above:

- They are not affected by the shape of the patient's face or the absence of teeth.
- The anaesthetist is not required to hold it in position or maintain a jaw thrust or chin lift thereby avoiding fatigue and allowing any other problems to be dealt with.
- They *significantly reduce* the risk of aspiration of regurgitated gastric contents but do not eliminate it completely.
- Their use is *relatively contraindicated* where there is an increased risk of regurgitation, for example in emergency cases, pregnancy and patients with a hiatus hernia.

In addition to the above, they have proved to be a valuable aid in those patients who are difficult to intubate, as they can usually be inserted to facilitate oxygenation while additional help or equipment is obtained (see below).

Insertion of a supraglottic airway (Fig. 4.8a–e)

The technique for insertion of an LMA is described, but the principles apply to all supraglottic devices, although not all have an inflatable cuff. The patient's reflexes must be suppressed to a level similar to that required for the insertion of

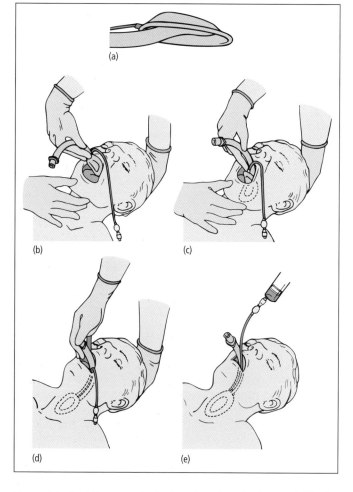

(a)

(b)

(c)

(d)

(e)

Figure 4.8 (a–e) Sequence for the insertion of a cuffed supraglottic airway device.

an oropharyngeal airway to prevent coughing or laryngospasm.

- The cuff is deflated (Fig. 4.8a) and the mask lightly lubricated.
- A head tilt is performed, the patient's mouth opened fully, and the tip of the mask inserted along the hard palate with the open side facing but not touching the tongue (Fig. 4.8b).
- The mask is further inserted, using the index finger to provide support for the tube (Fig. 4.8c). Eventually, resistance will be felt at the point where the tip of the mask lies at the upper oesophageal sphincter (Fig. 4.8d).
- The cuff is now fully inflated using an air-filled syringe attached to the valve at the end of the pilot tube (Fig. 4.8e).
- The laryngeal mask is secured either by a length of bandage or adhesive strapping attached to the protruding tube.
- A 'bite block' may be inserted to reduce the risk of damage to the LMA at recovery.

Tracheal intubation

This requires abolition of the laryngeal reflexes. During anaesthesia, this is achieved by giving a neuromuscular blocking drug. Alternatively, deep inhalational anaesthesia or local anaesthesia of the larynx can be used, but these are generally reserved for patients in whom difficulty with intubation is anticipated, for example in the presence of airway tumours or immobility of the cervical spine. The common indications for tracheal intubation are shown in Table 4.3.

Equipment for tracheal intubation

The equipment used will be determined by the circumstances and by the preferences of the individual anaesthetist. The following is a list of the basic needs for *adult oral* intubation:

- *Laryngoscope* with a curved (Macintosh) blade and functioning light.
- *Tracheal tubes (cuffed)* in a variety of sizes. The internal diameter is expressed in millimetres and the length in centimetres. They may be lightly lubricated.
  - *For males*: 8–9 mm internal diameter, 22–24 cm length.
  - *For females*: 7–8 mm internal diameter, 20–22 cm length.
- *Syringe* to inflate the cuff once the tube is in place.

Table 4.3 Common indications for tracheal intubation

- Where muscle relaxants are used to facilitate surgery (e.g. abdominal and thoracic surgery), thereby necessitating the use of mechanical ventilation.
- In patients with a full stomach, to protect against aspiration.
- Where the position of the patient would make airway maintenance difficult, e.g. the lateral or prone position.
- Where there is competition between surgeon and anaesthetist for the airway (e.g. operations on the head and neck).
- Where controlled ventilation is utilized to improve surgical access (e.g. neurosurgery).
- In those patients in whom the airway cannot be satisfactorily maintained by any other technique.
- During cardiopulmonary resuscitation.

- *Catheter mount*: to connect the tube to the anaesthetic system or ventilator tubing.
- *Suction*: switched on and immediately to hand in case the patient vomits or regurgitates.
- *Capnometer*: to detect carbon dioxide in expired gas (see below) thereby confirming placement of the tube in the airway.
- *Stethoscope*: to check ventilation of both lungs is occurring by listening for breath sounds during ventilation.
- *Extras*: a semi-rigid introducer to help mould the tube to a particular shape; Magill's forceps, designed to reach into the pharynx to remove debris or direct the tip of a tube; different size or style laryngoscope blade (for example, McCoy), bandage or tape to secure the tube.

The technique of oral intubation

Following IV induction, it is good practice to ensure that the patient can be ventilated via a facemask before giving the neuromuscular blocking drug to facilitate intubation. If intubation then proves to be unexpectedly difficult or impossible, the anaesthetist knows that oxygenation can be maintained and the patient will come to no harm. Along with the neuromuscular blocking drug, an IV opioid is often given to reduce the cardiovascular response to intubation. During the time it takes for a non-depolarizing neuromuscular blocker to reach maximal effect, there will be a period of apnoea. The patient will need to be ventilated manually with a mixture of oxygen and an inhalational drug to maintain anaesthesia. Once the degree of neuromuscular block is adequate, direct laryngoscopy is performed.

With the patient's head on a small pillow the neck is flexed and the head extended at the atlanto-occipital joint, the 'sniffing-the-morning-air' position. The patient's mouth is fully opened using the index finger and thumb of the *right* hand in a scissor action. The laryngoscope is held in the *left* hand and the blade introduced into the mouth along the right-hand side of the tongue, displacing it to the left. The blade is advanced until the tip lies in the gap between the base of the tongue and the epiglottis, the vallecula. Force is then applied *in the direction in which the handle of the laryngoscope is pointing*. The effort comes from the upper arm not the wrist, to lift the tongue and epiglottis. This exposes the larynx, seen as a triangular opening with the apex anteriorly and the whitish coloured true cords laterally (Fig. 4.9).

The tracheal tube is introduced into the right side of the mouth, advanced and seen to pass through the cords until the cuff lies just below them. The tube is then held firmly, the laryngoscope is carefully removed, and the cuff is inflated sufficiently to prevent any leak during ventilation. The patient is now ventilated manually while the position of the tube is confirmed, and it is secured to the patient using adhesive tape or cotton tape.

For some types of surgery, such as oral surgery, nasotracheal intubation is used so that the tube is out of the surgical field. A well-lubricated tube is introduced, usually via the right nostril, along the floor of the nose with the bevel pointing medially to avoid damage to the turbinates. It is advanced into the oro-pharynx, where it is usually visualized using a laryngoscope in the manner described above. It can then either be advanced directly into the larynx by pushing on the proximal end, or the tip picked up with Magill's forceps (which are designed not to impair the view of the larynx) and directed into the larynx. The procedure then continues as for oral intubation.

Confirming the position of the tracheal tube

Every tracheal tube inserted *must* have its position checked. This can be achieved using a number of techniques of varying reliability.

- *Measuring the carbon dioxide in expired gas (waveform capnometry):* The presence of carbon dioxide in expired gas indicates that the tube is in the airway, less than 0.2% indicates

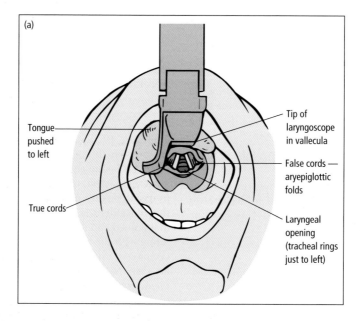

(a)

Tongue pushed to left

True cords

Tip of laryngoscope in vallecula

False cords — aryepiglottic folds

Laryngeal opening (tracheal rings just to left)

Figure 4.9 (a) Diagrammatic representation of the ideal view of the larynx at laryngoscopy.

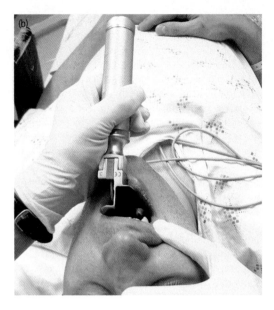

Figure 4.9 (b) Photograph showing tip of epiglottis during laryngoscopy.

oesophageal intubation. However, it does not indicate when the tube has been inserted too far and lies in a main bronchus. This can usually be determined by listening to both sides of the chest for equality of breath sounds.

- *Direct visualization:* Observing the tracheal tube passing between the vocal cords.
- *Oesophageal detector:* A 50 mL syringe is attached to the tracheal tube and the plunger rapidly withdrawn. If the tracheal tube is in the oesophagus, resistance is felt and air cannot be aspirated; if it is in the trachea, air is easily aspirated.
- *Fogging:* Seen on clear plastic tube connectors during expiration.
- *Less reliable signs are:*
  ○ diminished breath sounds on auscultation;
  ○ decreased chest movement on ventilation;
  ○ gurgling sounds over the epigastrium and 'burping' sounds as gas escapes;
  ○ a decrease in oxygen saturation detected by pulse oximetry. This occurs late, particularly if the patient has been preoxygenated.

Complications of tracheal intubation

The following complications are the more common ones, not an attempt to cover all eventualities.

Hypoxia, due to:

- *Unrecognized oesophageal intubation.* If there is any doubt about the position of the tube it should be removed and the patient ventilated via a facemask. This is most likely to occur when capnometry is unavailable.
- *Failed intubation and inability to ventilate the patient.* This is a rare event and usually a result of abnormal anatomy or airway pathology. In elective patients, it may be predictable at the preoperative assessment (see Chapter 1).
- *Failed ventilation after intubation.* Possible causes include the tube becoming kinked, blocked, disconnected, severe bronchospasm and tension pneumothorax. It may also be due to failure of the anaesthetic gas supply.
- *Aspiration.* Regurgitated gastric contents can cause blockage of the airways directly, or secondary to laryngeal spasm and bronchospasm. Cricoid pressure can be used to reduce the risk of regurgitation prior to intubation (see below).

Trauma:

- *Directly.* During laryngoscopy and insertion of the endotracheal tube, damage to lips, teeth, tongue, pharynx, larynx, trachea, and nose and nasopharynx during nasal intubation; causing soft tissue swelling or bleeding.
- *Indirectly.* To the recurrent laryngeal nerves, and the cervical spine and cord, particularly where there is pre-existing degenerative disease or trauma.

Reflex activity:

- *Hypertension and arrhythmias.* Occur in response to laryngoscopy and intubation and may jeopardize patients with coronary artery disease. In patients at risk, specific action is taken to attenuate the response – for example, pretreatment with beta blockers or potent analgesics (fentanyl, remifentanil).
- *Vomiting.* This may be stimulated when laryngoscopy is attempted in patients who are inadequately anaesthetised. It is more frequent when there is material in the stomach, as in emergencies when the patient is not starved, in patients with intestinal obstruction, or when gastric emptying is delayed, as after opiate analgesics or following trauma.
- *Laryngeal spasm.* Reflex adduction of the vocal cords as a result of stimulation of the epiglottis or larynx.

Keeping patients warm

NICE recommends that, following the induction of anaesthesia, a forced air-warming device should be used for all patients where anaesthesia is expected to last longer than 30 min to prevent intraoperative hypothermia. High-risk patients (ASA II to V, preoperative temperature <36 °C, general and regional anaesthesia, at risk of cardiovascular complications) should have forced air warming from the induction of anaesthesia, irrespective of the predicted duration. In addition, all fluids (particularly blood) should be warmed to 37 °C using a fluid warmer. Finally, inspired gases should be warmed and humidified and all non-surgical areas covered.

Maintenance of anaesthesia

The effects of the IV drug used for induction of anaesthesia wear off after a few minutes and unconsciousness must be maintained in some other way. This can be achieved using one of a variety of inhalational anaesthetics in oxygen with or without nitrous oxide, or by an intravenous infusion of a drug (TIVA), most commonly propofol. Whether the patient breathes spontaneously or is ventilated, the principles are similar.

Inhalational anaesthesia

The patient must receive an adequate:

- concentration of oxygen to prevent hypoxia;
- concentration of anaesthetic drug to ensure unconsciousness;
- flow of fresh gases to prevent hypercarbia.

In order to achieve these, the composition of the gas mixture is carefully monitored. The inspired oxygen concentration is usually maintained between 30 and 50%. This will be lower than the concentration being delivered by the anaesthetic machine when a circle system is being used because of the dilutional effect of the expired gases. The anaesthetic drug used is maintained at an appropriate end tidal concentration depending upon the patient, the surgical stimulus and the concurrent use of analgesic drugs.

In the spontaneously breathing patient, inadequate anaesthesia for the intensity of the surgical stimulus – for example, when surgery starts, will result in an increased respiratory rate and the patient may move as a result of reflex activity. In addition there may be an increase in heart rate and blood pressure. As a result the anaesthetist will increase the concentration of anaesthetic drug accordingly to deepen the level of unconsciousness. It may also be appropriate to halt surgery temporarily while this is achieved.

In the patient who has been given neuromuscular blocking drugs and is being ventilated, the anaesthetist must anticipate the need for changes in the depth of anaesthesia as the patient's ventilation will not change and they cannot move. Furthermore, if potent opioid analgesics have been given, changes in cardiovascular signs may be minimal. Consequently there is the possibility that the depth of anaesthesia is inadequate and the patient may be aware and unable to communicate this.

TIVA using propofol

With this technique, an appropriate brain concentration of propofol must be achieved and maintained to prevent awareness and any response to surgery. The simplest way is to give the usual IV induction dose, followed by repeated injections at intervals depending on the patient's response. This method can be used for short procedures, but for maintenance over a longer period it is more common to use a microprocessor-controlled infusion pump. This is more accurate and reliable as it uses the patient's weight and age to calculate the rate of infusion required to achieve a constant plasma (and brain) concentration. Having entered the appropriate data and started the pump, an initial rapid infusion is given to render the patient unconscious, followed by an infusion at a slower rate to maintain anaesthesia. This is often referred to as 'target controlled infusion' (TCI). The infusion rate, and hence plasma concentration, can also be adjusted manually to take account of individual patient variation and the degree of surgical stimulation in the same way that the concentration of an inhalational anaesthetic from the vaporizer can be changed.

Propofol alone can be used to maintain anaesthesia but the infusion rates required are very high, with significant cardiovascular side effects.

It is usually combined with IV opioids, either given as repeated injections (for example, fentanyl), or an infusion (for example, remifentanil). An alternative is to use a regional anaesthetic technique for analgesia. If muscle relaxation is required, neuromuscular blocking drugs are given and the patient is usually ventilated with oxygen-enriched air. Nitrous oxide can be used but this is not strictly TIVA and some of the advantages are lost.

Advantages of total intravenous anaesthesia

- The potential toxic effects of the inhalational anaesthetics are avoided.
- The problems associated with nitrous oxide can be avoided.
- A better quality of recovery is claimed.
- It may be beneficial in certain types of surgery, for example neurosurgery.
- Pollution is reduced.

Disadvantages of total intravenous anaesthesia

- Secure, reliable intravenous access is required.
- Risk of awareness if intravenous infusion fails.
- Cost of electronic infusion pumps.
- May cause profound hypotension.

Spontaneous ventilation

Theoretically any operation can be done with the patient breathing spontaneously. However, body cavity surgery, such as laparotomy, requires the inhibition of autonomic reflexes and significant muscle relaxation. This can only be achieved with relatively high concentrations of an inhaled or IV drug that result in respiratory depression or even apnoea. Furthermore, at the end of surgery, as high concentrations of drugs have been given, it will take longer to excrete or eliminate them, thereby prolonging the patient's recovery. Consequently, spontaneous ventilation is used predominantly for peripheral or body surface surgery, where minimal muscle relaxation is required and autonomic reflexes can be modified by the careful titration of small doses of IV opioids or the use of regional anaesthetic techniques.

Mechanical ventilation

The indications for using mechanical ventilation will vary amongst anaesthetists, but most would agree with using it in the following situations:

- where neuromuscular blocking drugs are used to facilitate surgical access, for example laparotomy;
- during thoracotomy to prevent paradoxical movement;
- when the anaesthetic technique will result in an unacceptable degree of respiratory depression;
- to allow control of carbon dioxide and cerebral blood flow during neurosurgery;
- during prolonged surgical procedures;
- surgery where intubation is required, for example prone surgery, full stomach, shared airway.

The anaesthetist will have to ensure that the correct ventilator settings are used for each patient to ensure adequate alveolar ventilation while minimizing the adverse effects of positive pressure. This will require setting of:

- tidal volume and respiratory rate or;
- minute volume and tidal volume – this will then determine respiratory rate;
- the mode of ventilation (volume or pressure controlled);
- the inspiratory and expiratory times;
- peak inspiratory pressure;
- the use of positive end expiratory pressure (PEEP) if required.

Modern ventilators have a range of integral monitors and alarms that can be set to indicate if the desired ventilation is not being achieved.

The effects of positive pressure ventilation

The reversal of the normal inspiratory pressure changes seen during mechanical ventilation has a number of important effects:

- There is an increase in the physiological dead space relative to the tidal volume and in ventilation/perfusion (V/Q) mismatch, both acting to impair oxygenation. An inspired oxygen concentration of at least 30% is used to compensate for this and prevent hypoxaemia.
- The $PaCO_2$ is dependent on alveolar ventilation. Hyperventilation results in hypocapnia, causing a respiratory alkalosis. This 'shifts' the oxyhaemoglobin dissociation curve to the left, increasing the affinity of haemoglobin for oxygen. Hypocapnia will induce vasoconstriction in

many organs, including the brain and heart, reducing blood flow. Underventilation will lead to hypercapnia, causing a respiratory acidosis. The effects on the oxyhaemoglobin dissociation curve are the opposite of the above, along with stimulation of the sympathetic nervous system causing vasodilatation, hypertension, tachycardia and arrhythmias.

- Excessive tidal volume may cause overdistension of the alveoli. In patients with pre-existing lung disease this may cause a pneumothorax and, if it continues long term, a condition called ventilator-induced lung injury.
- The positive intrathoracic pressure reduces venous return to the heart and cardiac output.
- Both systemic and pulmonary blood flow are reduced, the latter further increasing V/Q mismatch.

Transfer into the operating theatre

All of the above takes place in the anaesthetic room. At some point the patient has to be transferred into the operating theatre. This may take place with the patient already in position and on the operating table, or they may be taken into theatre on a trolley and then transferred onto the operating table. In either case, it will often mean disconnecting the patient from the anaesthesia machine and monitoring.

Once in theatre, the first manoeuvre must be to connect the patient to the breathing circuit and ensure that they are breathing or being ventilated adequately with an appropriate gas mixture. If not already on the operating table they are then transferred and the remaining monitoring attached. Every time a move has been completed it is essential to ensure that the airway is not compromised and ventilation maintained.

Positioning the patient

The patient is placed in a position to facilitate surgical access and there must always be sufficient theatre staff available to achieve this task safely, both for the patient and themselves. Some positions will require additional equipment; this must be assembled before any movement of the patient begins. The overall positioning is carried out

under the direction of, and with the assistance of, the anaesthetist. At all times the prime concern remains the safety of the patient. Detailed adjustment is carried out in conjunction with the surgeon.

The supine position (Fig. 4.10)

This position is used for the majority of surgical operations, but there is no room for complacency. The patient lies flat on their back, with their head and neck in a neutral position, unless the surgeon requires otherwise, for example for surgery to the ear. The arms are placed alongside the patient's sides or flexed at the elbow lying across the lower chest. If an arm or hand is to be operated on, this limb is usually abducted and supported on an arm table. The legs are extended in a neutral position.

In this position, the abdominal contents push the diaphragm into the thorax, reducing the lung volume, in particular the FRC. There is also the tendency for dependant alveoli to be better perfused but not as well ventilated. The overall effect is to reduce oxygenation of the blood, but this is compensated for by increasing the inspired oxygen concentration to a minimum of 30%

Points to note are as follows:

- the radial nerve is at risk from pressure midway along the humerus from a misplaced arm retainer;
- the ulnar nerve can be damaged at the elbow if allowed to lie over the edge of the mattress;
- the median nerve can be damaged in the antecubutal fossa by the distal edge of the blood pressure cuff if the elbow is flexed excessively;

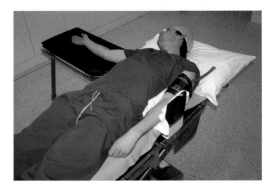

Figure 4.10   The supine position.

- the common peroneal nerve can be damaged by pressure against the head of the fibula;
- the head should be turned towards an abducted arm to reduce traction on the ipsilateral brachial plexus;
- pneumatic calf compression devices are used to reduce venous stasis in the legs and risk of deep venous thrombosis.

There are some variations in the supine position:

- *Trendelenburg.* Head down, using gravity to help displace bowels from the pelvis. Used in gynaecological and pelvic surgery.
- *Lithotomy.* With the hips and knees flexed to 90°, legs abducted slightly and the ankles supported in stirrups. Extremes of flexion and rotation must be avoided as the sciatic and femoral nerves can be damaged. The deep calf veins can be compressed against the stirrup poles. Used in gynaecological, urological and anorectal surgery.
- *Lloyd-Davies.* Hips and knees flexed 30–40°, abducted and supported in gutters. This position is designed to allow the surgical team combined access to the abdomen and perineum.

The lateral position (Fig. 4.11)

This is a relatively unstable position and requires a variety of additional supports to ensure the patient's safety. The anaesthetist takes responsibility for the patient's head, neck (and airway) and coordinates the team as the patient is turned. Depending on the site of surgery, (chest, abdomen (flank) or hip), supports are placed posteriorly against the pelvis, lumbar or thoracic spine and anteriorly against the iliac crests. The upper arm is usually supported in a small gutter, again the exact position depending on site of surgery, and the lower arm is placed to lie either across the chest or adjacent to the head, flexed at the shoulder and elbow.

In this position, during mechanical ventilation, the upper lung will be preferentially ventilated while the lower lung will receive a relatively greater blood flow. This can adversely affect oxygenation, particularly in patients with pre-existing pulmonary disease. More invasive monitoring may be used in this position.

There are some points to note:

- the patient's head and neck are supported to prevent traction on the brachial plexus on the uppermost side and a small support placed in the dependant axilla to prevent traction on the plexus on the patient's lower side;
- ensure that the patient's lower ear is not folded back on itself;
- the care when turning the patient to ensure that intravascular cannulas, tracheal tube and urinary catheter are not caught and removed.

The prone position (Fig. 4.12)

Many variations in this position have evolved using specially designed supports. Only the basic prone position will be described here.

As described above, the anaesthetist takes control of the head and neck and coordinates the team. With arms kept at the sides, the patient is

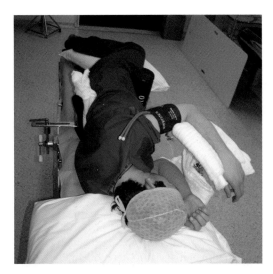

Figure 4.11 The lateral position.

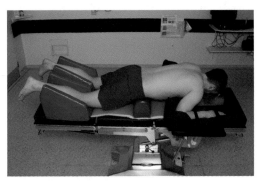

Figure 4.12 The prone position.

turned in two stages; firstly into the lateral position and then prone. It is essential that turning does not leave the patient flat on the table; either the head end of the table is lowered or the body raised to prevent excessive extension of the head and neck. Supports are required beneath the chest and pelvis, ensuring that the abdomen is free and the femoral vessels are not under undue pressure. The head must be supported in such a way as to prevent pressure on the eyes or tip of the nose, or occlusion of the tracheal tube. The patient's arms are either retained at the sides or flexed at the elbow and abducted at the shoulder to lie adjacent to their head. Finally, the knees are slightly flexed and padding is placed beneath the shins to raise the toes.

This position has the least detrimental effect on respiratory function. Ventilation and perfusion remain well matched, minimizing the risk of hypoxaemia. One of the main risks is obstruction of the inferior vena cava from badly placed supports reducing venous return, cardiac output and blood pressure. Careful checks must be made after turning the patient and close monitoring of the cardiovascular system is essential.

Points to note are:

- a reinforced tracheal tube is used to reduce the risk of the tube kinking – this would be difficult to correct once prone;
- great care must be taken with the cervical spine in *all* patients to prevent excessive rotation or extension;
- the arms must never be forced into position against resistance; the neck of the humerus is easily fractured;
- pressure on the eyes may cause thrombosis of the retinal artery and blindness;
- avoid compression of the femoral vessels in the groin; check the capillary refill time and colour of the feet after turning;
- ensure that pressure is not applied to the male genitalia by badly placed pelvic supports;
- avoid traction on the sciatic nerve by slightly flexing the knees;
- the abdomen must be free, particularly in spinal surgery, as compression of the inferior vena cava (IVC) will divert blood via the epidural veins that may compromise spinal surgery by excessive bleeding.

One of the commonest reasons for turning a surgical patient prone is to operate on the spine, as a result of degenerative disease processes or trauma, such as spinal fracture. As the patient will have normally been given neuromuscular blocking drugs, it is very easy to injure the spinal cord; either by placing the patient in an unsafe position or by uncontrolled or excessive movement when they are turned; the cervical spine is particularly susceptible. An experienced and fully coordinated team is essential when turning these patients.

Time out

Immediately before the start of the surgical intervention, the second stage of the WHO checklist is performed.

1 Confim that all the team members have introduced themselves by name and role.
2 The patient's identity must be confirmed, along with the planned procedure, side and site.
3 The anaesthetic, surgical and nursing teams should identify any anticipated problems, for example blood loss, equipment issues.
4 Antibiotic prophylaxis, glycaemic control and VTE prophylaxis have all been instituted where appropriate.
5 Imaging, for example X-rays and CT scans, is available and for the correct patient.

Once these have been confirmed and recorded, surgery can then start.

Assessment of neuromuscular blockade

The electrodes of the nerve stimulator can be applied to either the facial nerve just in front of the tragus or over the ulnar nerve at the wrist. A variety of sequences of electrical stimulation can be used to assess the intensity of neuromuscular block. This is useful during long surgical procedures, to control the timing of increments or adjust the rate of an infusion of neuromuscular blocking drugs to prevent coughing or sudden movement. This is particularly important during surgery in which a microscope is used, for example neurosurgery. At the end of surgery, it allows the anaesthetist to plan reversal of residual neuromuscular block to ensure adequate respiratory muscle function. It is also used to differentiate between apnoea due to prolonged action of suxamethonium, suggesting pseudocholinesterase deficiency, and residual non-depolarizing block, when both have been given. Finally, in recovery, the use of a nerve stimulator will allow the anaesthetist to distinguish between residual neuromuscular block and opioids overdose as a cause of inadequate ventilation postoperatively. The former will show reduced or absent response to stimulation, the latter a normal response.

Intraoperative fluids

The type and volume of fluid given during surgery varies for each and every patient, but must take into account:

- any deficit the patient has accrued;
- intraoperative requirements;
  - maintenance requirements during the procedure;
  - losses due to surgery;
- any vasodilatation secondary to the use of a regional anaesthetic technique (see Chapter 5).

The accrued deficit

This may be due to preoperative fasting, or losses as a result of vomiting, haemorrhage or pyrexia. Any deficit due to fasting is predominantly water from the total body water volume. The volume required is calculated at the normal daily maintenance rate of 1.5 mL/kg/h (from the point at which fasting began). Hartmann's solution is widely used intraoperatively rather than 0.9% saline to reduce the risk of hyperchloraemic acidosis. The other main cause of a preoperative deficit is losses either from or into the gastrointestinal tract. This fluid usually contains electrolytes and effectively depletes the extracellular volume. It is best replaced with a crystalloid of similar composition, particularly in respect of the sodium concentration; for example, 0.9% sodium chloride.

Acute blood loss preoperatively can be replaced with either an appropriate volume of crystalloid (remembering that only 30% remains intravascular) or colloid. If more than 30% of the estimated blood volume has been lost (approximately 1500 mL), and bleeding is ongoing, blood should be used.

Intraoperative requirements

Maintenance fluids are usually given when surgery is prolonged (along with any accrued deficit), or if there is the possibility of a delay in the patient resuming oral fluid intake. Most patients will compensate for a preoperative deficit by increasing their oral intake postoperatively. When maintenance fluid is used it should be given at 1.5 mL/kg/h, and increased if the patient is pyrexial by 10% for each degree centigrade above normal.

Losses during surgery are due to:

- *Evaporation:* this can occur during body cavity surgery or when large areas of tissue are exposed, depleting the total body water.
- *Trauma:* leads to the formation of tissue oedema, the volume of which is dependent upon the extent of tissue damage. This fluid is similar in composition to extracellular fluid and is often referred to as 'third-space loss' (see Chapter 7). Third-space fluids are not of any functional use to the body, and lead to a deficit in the ECF volume.
- *Blood loss:* this will depend upon the type and site of surgery.

Fluid losses from the first two causes are difficult to measure and are extremely variable. If evaporative losses are considered excessive, then 4% glucose plus 0.18% saline can be used. Third-space losses should be replaced with a solution similar in composition to extracellular fluid, and Hartmann's is commonly used. The rate fluid is given and volume required is proportional to surgical trauma and may be as much as 10 mL/kg/h. Blood pressure, pulse, peripheral perfusion and urine output will give an indication as to the adequacy of replacement. However, in complex cases (major abdominal, urological and orthopaedic surgery) there is now evidence that patients whose fluid status is managed using the information provided by using an oesophageal Doppler to monitor stroke volume and cardiac output, have better outcomes.

Blood loss is slightly more obvious and can be estimated by weighing surgical swabs and noting the volume in the suction apparatus (minus the volume of any saline washes used). Most, previously well patients will tolerate the anaemia that results from the loss of 30% of their blood volume, providing that the circulating volume is adequately maintained by the use of crystalloids or colloids. Beyond this, red cell preparations are used in order to maintain the oxygen-carrying capacity of the blood. A haemoglobin level between 8 and 10 g/dL is safe even for those patients with serious cardiorespiratory disease. In most cases, the equivalent of the patient's estimated blood volume can be replaced with red cell concentrates, crystalloid and colloid in the appropriate volumes. Occasionally blood loss is such that the haemostatic mechanisms are affected, for example after major trauma or vascular injury. This may be seen as continuous oozing from the surgical wound or around IV cannulation sites. Most hospitals now have a 'massive transfusion protocol', which is triggered either by loss of one blood volume (estimated as 70 mL/kg) or ongoing bleeding at a rate of >150 mL/min. Blood should be taken for haemoglobin concentration, platelet count, prothrombin time, (PT or INR), fibrinogen levels and treatment should begin empirically with further units of packed cells supplemented with fresh frozen plasma and platelets in approximately a 1:1:1 ratio. Consideration may also be given to the use of tranexamic acid and recombinant factor VIIa.

The anaesthetic record

On every occasion an anaesthetic is given, a comprehensive and *legible* record must be made. The details and method of recording will vary with each case, the type of chart used and the equipment available. The anaesthetic record is valuable to future anaesthetists who encounter the patient, particularly when there has been a difficulty (for example, with intubation), and is also a medicolegal document, which may be referred to after several years. An anaesthetic chart typically allows the following to be recorded:

- preoperative findings, ASA grade, premedication;
- details of previous anaesthetics and any difficulties;
- apparatus used for the current anaesthetic;
- monitoring devices used;
- anaesthetic and other drugs given: timing, dose and route;
- vital signs at various intervals, usually depicted graphically;
- fluids given and lost: type and volume;
- use of local or regional anaesthetic techniques;
- anaesthetic difficulties or complications;
- postoperative instructions.

Increasingly, electronic records are being developed. These have the advantage of allowing the anaesthetist to concentrate on caring for the patient, particularly during an emergency, rather than having to stop and make a record or try to fill in the record retrospectively.

Emergence from anaesthesia

Sign out

When the surgical procedure has been completed and before any member of the team leaves the operating theatre, a number of final checks are made:

1 Confirmation that all instruments, swabs are complete and accounted for.
2 All specimens are correctly labelled.
3 The procedure has been recorded accurately.
4 Have any equipment issues been identified that need addressing?
5 Are there any concerns for the immediate recovery and postoperative management for the patient?

Once these have been completed, the anaesthetist has to reverse the process of anaesthesia, often referred to as 'waking the patient up'. As a consequence of the wide variety of anaesthetic techniques used, there is no absolute protocol for this stage of anaesthesia. However, there are two main priorities – recovery of consciousness and maintenance of a patent airway. Here, these will be described in relation to patients breathing spontaneously and those being ventilated.

1. Spontaneous ventilation, inhalational drug for maintenance, supraglottic airway

At the end of surgery, the vaporizer is turned off and the patient allowed to eliminate the inhaled anaesthetic. If a circle system is being used the patient will continue to rebreathe the exhaled gas. This will contain some anaesthetic agent and so the alveolar and hence plasma concentrations will only fall very slowly, delaying recovery. Therefore, to speed up elimination of the anaesthetic, the flow of oxygen into the circle is increased to around 10–15 L/min. This excess flow flushes exhaled gas out of the circle, rebreathing is eliminated and the inspired oxygen concentration is almost 100%. The supraglottic airway will now need to be removed. There are two options as to when this is done:

- Leave it in place with the patient breathing oxygen until laryngeal reflexes have been restored.

The disadvantage to this is that occasionally it may result in the patient biting on the tube and obstructing the airway.

- Remove while deeply unconscious. This is easier but leaves the airway unprotected and the lack of muscle tone may result in airway obstruction and the need for the anaesthetist to perform a chin lift or jaw thrust.

Once the device has been removed, oxygen is given via a facemask and, if not already carried out, the patient is transferred from the operating table onto a trolley or bed. As patients begin to obey commands they can be sat up at 30° if it is safe to do so.

2. Mechanical ventilation, inhalational drug for maintenance, tracheal tube

The main difference from what has already been described is that normal neuromuscular function has to be restored before the patient regains consciousness. Therefore, recovery needs to be coordinated with the point at which the neuromuscular blocking drug wears off spontaneously or is antagonized. This is best checked by using a peripheral nerve stimulator. As before, the fresh gas flow is increased and the patient ventilated with 100% oxygen to eliminate the volatile drug. If necessary a dose of neostigmine (2.5 mg) is given to antagonize the effect of the neuromuscular blocker. This is given along with an anticholinergic, usually glycopyrrolate, to block the unwanted muscarinic effects of neostigmine. The aim is to restore spontaneous ventilation before removal of the tracheal tube. Once ventilation commences, a similar dilemma over when to remove the tube is encountered as before.

- Remove the tube while the patient is deeply unconscious. This leaves the airway unprotected and at risk of obstruction and the need for support by the anaesthetist or the use of an oropharyngeal airway. Furthermore there is also the risk of the patient developing laryngospasm if any soiling of the larynx occurs (for example, from saliva or regurgitated gastric contents) as the patient recovers.
- Leave the tube in place until the patient is nearly conscious. Apart from the risk of occlusion by the patient biting the tube, the presence of the tube may also induce severe coughing and breath holding by the patient. This may cause hypoxia, as well as being painful after abdominal surgery, and

undesirable after intracranial surgery as it may precipitate bleeding.

When a TIVA technique has been used to maintain anaesthesia, the principles are the same, except that the infusions are stopped to allow the plasma concentration of drug to fall to promote diffusion out of the brain. When remifentanil has been used intraoperatively, the patient will need to be given an alternative analgesic before recovering to prevent severe pain on awakening.

FURTHER USEFUL INFORMATION

Allman KG, Wilson IH (eds) *Oxford handbook of anaesthesia*, 3rd edn. Oxford: Oxford University Press, 2011

Cook TM, Woodall N, Frerk C. Fourth National Audit Project. Major complications of airway management in the UK: results of the Fourth National Audit Project of the Royal College of Anaesthetists. *British Journal of Anaesthesia* 2011; **106**: 266–71

McGrath CD, Hunter JM. Monitoring of neuromuscular block. continuing education in anaesthesia. *Critical Care and Pain* 2006; **6**(1): 7–12.

Spoors C, Kiff K (eds). *Training in anaesthesia*. Oxford: Oxford University Press, 2010.

www.aagbi.org/publications/guidelines/docs/anaesthesiateam05.pdf
[The anaesthesia team. Revised edition 2005. The Association of Anaesthetists of Great Britain & Ireland.]

www.aagbi.org/publications/guidelines/docs/checking04.pdf
[Checking anaesthetic equipment. The Association of Anaesthetists of Great Britain & Ireland.2004.]

http://anestit.unipa.it/HomePage.html
[The best anaesthesia site on the web, with free sign-on. A virtual textbook of anaesthesia that includes a good section on airway management.]

www.carg.cochrane.org/en/index.html
[This site contains systematic reviews of aspects of anaesthetic practice.]

www.das.uk.com/
[The Difficult Airway Society website contains guidance on management of airway emergencies including failed intubation drills.]

www.nice.org.uk/CG65
[Guidelines from NICE on the prevention of perioperative hypothermia.]

www.nice.org.uk/pdf/Ultrasound_49_GUID-ANCE.pdf

[Guidance from the National Institute of Clinical Excellence (NICE) on the use of ultrasound locating devices for placing central venous catheters.]

www.nrls.npsa.nhs.uk/resources/?
EntryId45=59860

[The National Patient Safety Agency (NPSA) website with details of the World Health Organisation Surgical Safety Checklist implemented in 2009.]

www.rcoa.ac.uk/docs/tiva_info.pdf

[A report from the Safe Anaesthesia Liason Group, with recommendations for ensuring drug delivery during TIVA, 2009.]

www.reducinglengthofstay.org.uk/doc/isog_report.pdf

[Improving surgical outcome group. Interesting report on how outcomes after major surgery can be improved.]

All websites last accessed February 2012.

? SELF-ASSESSMENT

Short-answer questions

4.1 What are the main advantages and disadvantages of inhalational induction of anaesthesia?

4.2 List, in order of reliability, the checks that can be performed to confirm the position of a tracheal tube. Give five common complications of tracheal intubation.

4.3 Give an example of a total intravenous anaesthetic technique (TIVA) in a patient undergoing a laparotomy. Give four potential advantages and four disadvantages of this technique.

4.4 What are common indications for ventilating a patient during surgery? What are the potential adverse effects of using this technique?

4.5 What factors are taken into account when calculating intraoperative fluid requirements? How much intraoperative fluid would you expect to give to an 80 kg man having a total hip replacement at 09:00 under general anaesthesia? He has been fasting since 03:00, surgery takes 90 min and blood loss is approximately 600 ml. Would having a spinal anaesthetic make any difference to his requirements and if so by how much?

4.6 What are the three stages of the Surgical Safety Checklist? What is checked at each stage?

True/false questions

4.1 The following are essential monitors during anaesthesia:
a ECG;
b non-invasive blood pressure;
c temperature;
d pulse oximetry.

4.2 Oesophageal intubation can be confirmed rapidly using:
a pulse oximetry;
b waveform capnometry;
c auscultation for breath sounds during ventilation;
d visualization of the tube passing through the cords.

4.3 During general anaesthesia:
a mechanical ventilation will be required for all procedures lasting longer than 30 min;
b there is an increase in the patient's functional residual capacity (FRC);
c there is an increase in ventilation/perfusion mismatch;
d mechanical ventilation improves venous return to the heart helping maintain cardiac output.

4.4 Intraoperatively:
a evaporation of fluid during a laparotomy can cause significant loss;
b when maintenance fluids are required, these should be given at a rate of 1.5 mL/kg/h;
c up to 50% blood volume can be lost before transfusion is required;
d the use of large volumes of 0.9% (normal) saline may cause hyperchloraemic alkalosis.

4.5 When positioning the patient for surgery:
a the radial nerve can be injured occur at the medial epicondyle of the humerus;
b in the lateral position the brachial plexus can be subject to stretch on both sides of the neck;
c when one arm is abducted, the patient's head should be turned towards the same side;
d respiratory function is not compromised in the Trendelenberg position.

Local and regional anaesthesia

When referring to local and regional techniques and the drugs used, the terms 'analgesia' and 'anaesthesia' are used loosely and interchangeably. For clarity and consistency the following terms will be used:

- *Analgesia:* the state when only relief of pain is provided. This may allow some minor surgical procedures to be performed. An example is infiltration analgesia for suturing.
- *Anaesthesia:* the state when analgesia is accompanied by muscle relaxation, usually to allow major surgery to be undertaken. Regional anaesthesia may be used alone or in combination with general anaesthesia.

The role of local and regional anaesthesia

Regional anaesthesia is not just an answer to the problem of anaesthesia in patients regarded as not well enough for general anaesthesia. The decision to use any of these techniques should be based on the advantages offered to both the patient and surgeon. The following are some of the considerations taken into account:

- analgesia or anaesthesia is provided predominantly in the area required, thereby avoiding the systemic effects of drugs;
- spontaneous ventilation can be preserved and respiratory depressant drugs avoided in patients with chronic respiratory disease;
- there is generally less disturbance of the control of coexisting systemic disease requiring medical therapy, such as diabetes mellitus;
- the airway reflexes are preserved and, in a patient with a full stomach, particularly due to delayed gastric emptying (for example, in pregnancy), the risk of aspiration is reduced;
- central neural blockade may improve access and facilitate surgery, for example by causing contraction of the bowel or by providing profound muscle relaxation;
- blood loss can be reduced with controlled hypotension;
- there is a considerable reduction in the equipment required and the cost of anaesthesia – this may be important in underdeveloped areas;

- when used in conjunction with general anaesthesia, only sufficient anaesthetic (inhalational or IV) is required to maintain unconsciousness, with analgesia and muscle relaxation provided by the regional technique;
- some techniques can be continued postoperatively to provide pain relief, for example an epidural;
- complications after major surgery, particularly orthopaedic surgery, are significantly reduced.

> A patient should never be forced to accept a local or regional technique. Initial objections and fears are best alleviated, and usually overcome, by explanation of the advantages and by reassurance.

Whenever a local or regional anaesthetic technique is used, facilities for resuscitation must always be immediately available in order that allergic reactions and toxicity can be dealt with effectively. As a minimum this will include the following:

- equipment to maintain and secure the airway, give oxygen and provide ventilation;
- intravenous cannulas and a range of fluids;
- drugs, including adrenaline, atropine, vasopressors and anticonvulsants;
- suction;
- a surface for the patient that is capable of being tipped head-down.

Local and regional anaesthetic techniques

Local anaesthetics can be used:

- topically to a mucous membrane, such as the eye or urethra;
- for subcutaneous infiltration;
- intravenously after the application of a tourniquet (IVRA);
- directly around nerves, for example the brachial plexus;
- in the extradural space ('epidural anaesthesia');
- in the subarachnoid space ('spinal anaesthesia').

The latter two techniques are more correctly called 'central neural blockade'; however, the term 'spinal anaesthesia' is commonly used when local anaesthetic is injected into the subarachnoid space and it is in this context that it will be used. The following is a brief introduction to some of the more popular regional anaesthetic techniques; those who require more detail should consult the texts in 'further useful information'.

Infiltration analgesia (Fig. 5.1)

Lidocaine 0.5% is used for short procedures, for example suturing a wound, and 0.5% bupivacaine or chirocaine for pain relief from a surgical incision. A solution containing adrenaline can be used if a large dose or a prolonged effect is required, providing that tissues around end arteries are avoided. Infiltration analgesia is not instantaneous and lack of patience is the commonest reason for failure. The technique used is as follows:

1. Calculate the maximum volume of drug that can be used (see Chapter 3).
2. Clean the skin surrounding the wound with an appropriate solution and allow it to dry.
3. Insert the needle subcutaneously, avoiding any obvious blood vessels.
4. Aspirate to ensure that the tip of the needle does not lie in a blood vessel. If blood is aspirated discard the syringe and start again.
5. Inject the local anaesthetic in a constant flow as the needle is withdrawn. Too rapid injection will cause pain.
6. Second and subsequent punctures should be made through an area of skin already anaesthetised.

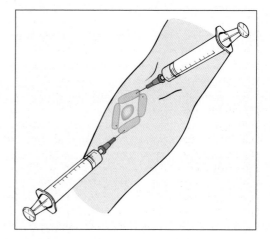

Figure 5.1   Infiltration with local anaesthetic.

In a clean wound, local anaesthetic can be injected directly into the exposed wound edge. This technique can also be used at the end of surgery to help reduce wound pain postoperatively.

Brachial plexus block

The nerves of the brachial plexus can be anaesthetised by injecting the local anaesthetic drug either above the level of the clavicle (supraclavicular approach or interscalene approach) or where they enter the arm through the axilla along with the axillary artery and vein (axillary approach). A nerve stimulator is used to locate the nerves and increasingly ultrasound is also being used allow more precise insertion of the needle and avoid nerve injury and intravascular injection of the local anaesthetic drug. All of the drugs in Table 3.10 can be used. These techniques can be used for a wide range of surgical procedures; interscalene blocks are used for shoulder surgery whereas an axillary block is useful for operations below the elbow. Both will provide good analgesia in the immediate postoperative period. The block may last several hours, and so it is important to warn both the surgeon and patient of this.

Transversus abdominis plane (TAP) block

As the name suggests, this block aims to deposit local anaesthetic in the plane between the transversus abdominis and internal oblique muscles (Fig. 5.2a) to anaesthetise the nerves supplying the skin and muscles of the anterior abdominal wall (and parietal peritoneum). Although the block can be performed blind using anatomical landmarks, ultrasound guidance is increasingly used to locate the correct plane between the muscles. The needle is inserted in the midaxillary line midway between the costal margin and iliac crest. When the needle reaches the correct plane, 2–3 ml saline is injected to confirm the location, followed by the local anaesthetic (Fig. 5.2b). Alternatively, a catheter can be inserted and an infusion of local anaesthetic given for prolonged analgesia. For midline incisions, bilateral blocks will be required and care must be taken not to exceed the maximum safe dose of local anaesthetic. The block is most useful in lower abdominal surgery, for example appendicectomy, hernia repair, abdominal hysterectomy, operations on the kidney and laparoscopic surgery.

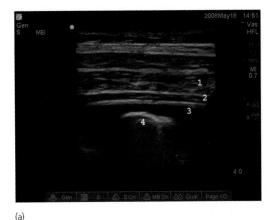

(a)

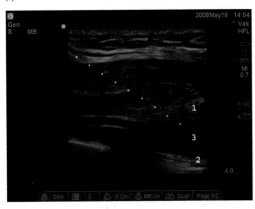

(b)

Figure 5.2 (a) Ultrasound image of anatomy for TAP block. 1; internal oblique, 2; transverses abdominis, 3; peritoneal cavity, 4; bowel. (b) Ultrasound image of TAP block. 1; internal oblique, 2; displaced transverses abdominis, 3; pool of local anaesthetic solution. Dotted line indicates position of needle. *(Courtesy Dr J Corcoran).*

Epidural anaesthesia

Epidural (extradural) anaesthesia involves the deposition of a local anaesthetic drug into the potential space *outside* the dura (Fig. 5.3a). This space extends from the craniocervical junction at C1 to the sacrococcygeal membrane, and anaesthesia can theoretically be safely instituted at any level in between. In practice, an epidural is sited adjacent to the nerve roots that supply the surgical site; that is, the lumbar region is used for pelvic and lower limb surgery and the thoracic region for abdominal surgery. A single injection of local anaesthetic can be given, but more commonly a catheter is inserted into the epidural space and either

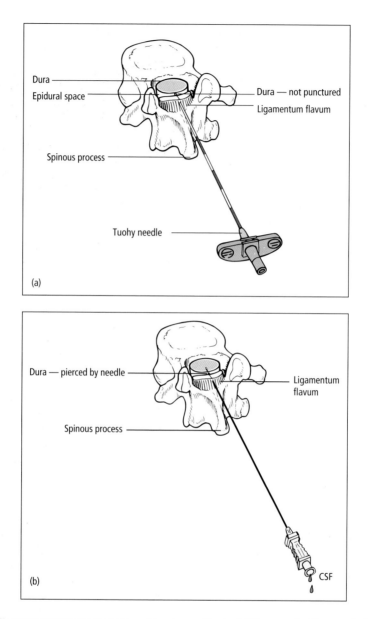

(a)

(b)

CSF

Figure 5.3 (a) Placement of the needle tip for epidural anaesthesia. (b) Placement of the needle tip for spinal (intrathecal) anaesthesia. From Gwinnutt CL *Clinical Anaesthesia*. Oxford: Blackwell Science, 1996.

repeated injections or a constant infusion of a local anaesthetic drug is used.

To aid identification of the epidural space, a technique termed 'loss of resistance' is used. The (Tuohy) needle is advanced until its tip is embedded within the ligamentum flavum (yellow ligament). This blocks the tip and causes marked resistance to attempted injection of either air or saline from a syringe attached to the needle. As the needle is advanced further, the ligament is pierced, resistance disappears dramatically and air or saline is injected easily. The needle has markings every 1 cm to enable determination of the depth of the epidural space.

A plastic catheter is then inserted into the epidural space via the needle. The catheter is marked at 5 cm intervals to 20 cm with extra markings every 1 cm between 5 and 15 cm. Knowing how far the catheter has been inserted, as well as the depth of the epidural space, allows calculation of the length of the catheter in the epidural space.

Varying concentrations of local anaesthetics are used depending on what effect is required. When using bupivacaine or chirocaine, 0.5% will be needed for surgical anaesthesia with muscle relaxation, but only 0.1–0.2% for postoperative analgesia. Local anaesthetic will spread from the level of injection both up and down the epidural space. The extent of anaesthesia is determined by:

- The spinal level of insertion of the epidural. For a given volume, spread is greater in the thoracic region than in the lumbar region.
- The volume of local anaesthetic injected.
- Gravity: tipping the patient head-down encourages spread cranially, while head-up tends to limit spread.

The spread of anaesthesia is described with reference to the limits of the dermatomes affected; for example, the inguinal ligament, T12; the umbilicus, T10; and the nipples, T4. An opioid is often given with the local anaesthetic to improve the quality and duration of analgesia, for instance fentanyl 50 µg. For details of infusions of local anaesthetics and opioids for postoperative analgesia, see Chapter 7.

Spinal anaesthesia

Spinal (intrathecal) anaesthesia results from the injection of a local anaesthetic drug directly into the cerebrospinal fluid (CSF) within the subarachnoid space (Fig. 5.3b). The spinal needle can only be inserted below the second lumbar and above the first sacral vertebrae; the upper limit is determined by the termination of the spinal cord and the lower limit by the fact that the sacral vertebrae are fused and access becomes virtually impossible. A single injection of local anaesthetic is normally used, thereby limiting the duration of the technique.

A fine, 22–29 g needle with a 'pencil point' or tapered point (for example, a Whitacre or Sprotte needle) is used (Fig. 5.4). The small diameter and shape are an attempt to reduce the incidence of

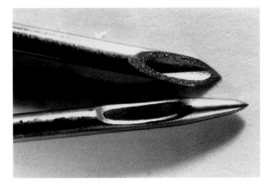

Figure 5.4 Photomicrograph showing the shape of a bevel needle (*top*) and 'pencil point' needle (*below*). From Jones MJ, Selby IR, Gwinnutt CL Hughes DG. Technical note: the influence of using an atraumatic needle on the incidence of post-myelography headache. *British Journal of Radiology* 1994; **67**: 396–98.

post dural puncture headache (see below). To aid passage of this needle through the skin and interspinous ligament, a short, wide-bore needle is introduced initially and the spinal needle passed through its lumen.

Factors influencing the spread of the local anaesthetic drug within the CSF, and hence the extent of anaesthesia, include:

- Use of hyperbaric solutions (its specific gravity is greater than that of CSF), for example 'heavy' bupivacaine (0.5%). This is achieved by the addition of 8% dextrose. Posture is then used to control spread.
- Positioning of the patient either during or after the injection. Maintenance of the sitting position after injection results in a block of the low lumbar and sacral nerves. In the supine position, the block will extend to the thoracic nerves around T5–6, the point of maximum backwards curve (kyphosis) of the thoracic spine. Further extension can be obtained with a head-down tilt.
- Increasing the dose (volume and/or concentration) of local anaesthetic drug.
- The higher the placement of the spinal anaesthetic in the lumbar region, the higher the level of block obtained.

Small doses of an opioid, for example morphine or diamorphine 0.1–0.25 mg, may be injected with the local anaesthetic. This extends the duration of analgesia for up to 12 hours postoperatively.

Contraindications to epidural and spinal anaesthesia

Hypovolaemia: either as a result of blood loss or dehydration. Such patients are likely to experience severe falls in cardiac output as compensatory vasoconstriction is lost.

A low, fixed cardiac output: as seen with severe aortic or mitral stenosis. The reduced venous return further reduces cardiac output, jeopardizing perfusion of vital organs.

Local skin sepsis: risk of introducing infection.

Coagulopathy: either as a result of a bleeding diathesis (for example, haemophilia) or therapeutic anticoagulation. This risks causing an epidural haematoma. There may also be a very small risk in patients taking aspirin and associated drugs that reduce platelet activity. Where heparins are used perioperatively to reduce the risk of deep venous thrombosis, these may be started after the insertion of the epidural or spinal.

Raised intracranial pressure: a risk of precipitating coning.

Known allergy to amide local anaesthetic drugs.

A patient who is totally uncooperative.

Concurrent disease of the CNS: some would caution against the use of these techniques for fear of being blamed for any subsequent deterioration.

Previous spinal surgery or abnormal spinal anatomy: although not an absolute contraindication, epidural or spinal anaesthesia may be technically difficult.

Monitoring during local and regional anaesthesia

During epidural and spinal anaesthesia, the guidelines on monitoring (see Chapter 4) should be followed. A conscious patient is not an excuse for inadequate monitoring! Particular attention must be paid to the cardiovascular system as a result of the profound effects these techniques can have. Maintenance of verbal contact with the patient is useful as it gives an indication of cerebral perfusion. Early signs of inadequate cardiac output are complaints of nausea and faintness, and subsequent vomiting. The first indication of extensive spread of anaesthesia may be a complaint of difficulty with breathing or numbness in the fingers. Clearly, these valuable signs and symptoms will be lost if the patient is heavily sedated.

Complications of central neural blockade

These are usually mild and rarely cause any lasting morbidity (Table 5.1). Those commonly seen intraoperatively are predominantly due to the effects of the local anaesthetic. Their management is covered below. Complications seen in patients receiving epidural analgesia postoperatively are covered in Chapter 7.

Hypotension and bradycardia

Anaesthesia of the lumbar and thoracic nerves causes progressive sympathetic block, causing vasodilatation and a reduction in the peripheral resistance and venous return to the heart and so cardiac output falls. If the block extends cranially beyond T5, the cardioaccelerator nerves are also blocked, and the unopposed vagal tone results in a bradycardia. Small falls in blood pressure are tolerated and may be helpful in reducing blood loss. If the blood pressure falls by >25% of resting value, or the patient becomes symptomatic (see below), treatment consists of:

- oxygen via a facemask;
- IV fluids (crystalloids or colloids) to increase venous return;
- vasopressors to counteract the vasodilatation, either ephedrine, an α- and β-agonist (3 mg IV) or metaraminol, an α -agonist (0.25 mg IV);
- atropine 0.5 mg IV to counteract bradycardia.

Nausea and vomiting

These are most often the first indications of hypotension and cerebral hypoxia but can also result from vagal stimulation during upper abdominal surgery. Any hypotension or hypoxia is corrected as described above. If due to surgery, try to reduce

Table 5.1 **Incidence of common complications with spinal anaesthesia**

• Hypotension	33%
• Nausea	18%
• Bradycardia	13%
• Vomiting	7%
• Dysrhythmias	2%
• Post dural puncture headache	<1%

the degree of manipulation. If this is not possible then it may be necessary to convert to general anaesthesia. Atropine 0.3–0.6 mg is frequently effective, particularly if there is a bradycardia. Anti-emetics can be tried (for example, ondansetron 4 mg IV), but this must not be at the expense of the above.

Post dural puncture headache

Caused by a persistent leak of CSF from the needle hole in the dura. The incidence is greatest with large holes – that is, when a hole is made accidentally during epidural anaesthesia, and least after spinal anaesthesia using fine needles (for example 26 g) with a pencil or tapered point (<1%). Patients usually complain of a headache that is frontal or occipital, postural and exacerbated by straining. The majority will resolve spontaneously. Persistent headaches can be relieved (>90%) by injecting 20–30 mL of the patient's own venous blood into the epidural space (epidural blood patch) under strict aseptic conditions.

Local anaesthetic toxicity

This is usually the result of one of the following:

- *Rapid absorption of a normally safe dose.* Use of an excessively concentrated solution or injection into a vascular area results in rapid absorption. It can also occur during intravenous regional anaesthesia (IVRA – see below) if the tourniquet is released too soon or accidentally.
- *Inadvertent IV injection.* failure to aspirate prior to injection via virtually any route.
- *Overdose.* Failure or error in either calculating the maximum safe dose or taking into account any pre-existing cardiac or hepatic disease.

Signs and symptoms of toxicity are due to effects on the central nervous system and the cardiovascular system. These are dependent on the plasma concentration and initially may represent either a mild toxicity or, more significantly, the early stages of a more severe reaction:

- *Mild or early.* Circumoral paraesthesia, numbness of the tongue, visual disturbances, lightheadedness, slurred speech, twitching, restlessness, mild hypotension and bradycardia.

- *Severe or late.* Grand mal convulsions followed by coma, respiratory depression and eventually apnoea, cardiovascular collapse with profound hypotension and bradycardia, and ultimately cardiac arrest.

The incidence of severe systemic toxicity varies from 1 in 1000 with peripheral nerve blocks to 1 in 10 000 with epidural anaesthesia

Management of toxicity

If a patient complains of any of the above symptoms or exhibits signs, stop giving the local anaesthetic immediately! The next steps consist of:

- *Airway:* maintain using basic techniques. Tracheal intubation will be needed if the protective reflexes are absent to protect against aspiration.
- *Breathing:* give oxygen (100%) with support of ventilation if inadequate.
- *Circulation:* raise the patient's legs to encourage venous return and start an IV infusion of crystalloid or colloid. Treat a bradycardia with IV atropine.
- *Disability:* convulsions must be treated early. Diazepam 5–10 mg intravenously can be used initially but this may cause significant respiratory depression. If the convulsions do not respond or they recur, then seek assistance.

Circulatory collapse

Recently, anecdotal evidence strongly suggests that the use of lipid solutions given intravenously improve the outcome when local anaesthetic toxicity causes profound circulatory collapse and cardiac arrest. In such circumstances, the AAGBI have issued the following guidelines:

- start cardiopulmonary resuscitation (CPR) using current guidelines;
- manage any arrhythmias according to current protocols;
- start IV lipid emulsion therapy:
  - give 1.5 mL/kg 20% lipid emulsion (approx 100 ml) over 1 min;
  - start an infusion of 20% lipid emulsion at a rate of 15 mL/kg/h;
- after 5 min, if cardiovascular stability has not been restored or an adequate circulation deteriorates:
  - repeat two boluses, 5 min apart;
  - double the rate of the infusion;
- do not exceed a maximum dose of 12 mL/kg.

If resuscitation is ongoing or successful, the patient should be transferred to a critical care area. The patient should be monitored for at least 48 hours for the development of pancreatitis and the case should be reported to www.lipidregistry.org.

Because of the risk of an inadvertent overdose of a local anaesthetic drug, they should only be given where full facilities for monitoring and resuscitation are immediately available. This ensures the maximum chance of patient recovery without any permanent sequelae.

Regional anaesthesia: in awake or anaesthetised patients?

Major nerve blocks and epidural anaesthesia are often combined with general anaesthesia to reduce the amount and number of systemic drugs given, and to provide postoperative analgesia. Claimed advantages of performing the block with the patient awake are:

- the block can be checked before surgery commences to ensure it works satisfactorily;
- the risk of nerve injury is reduced as the patient will complain if the needle touches a nerve;
- the patient can cooperate with positioning.

Advantages claimed for performing the block after induction of anaesthesia are:

- it is more pleasant for the patient, with no discomfort during insertion of the needle;
- there is no risk of the patient suddenly moving;
- it allows easier positioning of patients in pain, for example due to fractures;

- if the needle hits the nerve then the damage has already been done.

Fortunately, in experienced hands with either technique, the risk of nerve injury resulting in permanent sequelae is very rare. However, all patients who have a regional technique should be assessed to ensure that there is full recovery of normal function.

FURTHER USEFUL INFORMATION

Fischer HBJ, Pinnock CA (eds) *Fundamentals of regional anaesthesia.* Cambridge: Cambridge University Press, 2004.

Nicholls B, Conn D, Roberts A. *The Abbott pocket guide to practical peripheral nerve blockade.* Maidenhead: Abbott Anaesthesia, 2008.

Spoors C, Kiff K (eds) *Training in anaesthesia.* Oxford: Oxford University Press, 2010.

http://www.aagbi.org/sites/default/files/la_toxicity_2010_0.pdf
[Downloadable chart for management of severe local anaesthetic toxicity.]

www.lipidrescue.squarespace.com
[Dedicated site to improving knowledge on the use of lipid to treat cardiac toxicity following local anaesthetic overdose.]

http://www.nysora.com/
[The best regional anaesthesia website.]

http://www.oxsora.com/
[Website with useful video clips of blocks being performed under ultrasound.]

http://www.rcoa.ac.uk/index.asp?PageID=717
[The report of a national Audit project looking into the complications of neuraxial block in the UK, 2009.]

All websites last accessed February 2012.

? SELF-ASSESSMENT

Short-answer questions

5.1 What are the potential benefits of regional anaesthesia?

5.2 What are the contraindications to performing epidural and spinal anaesthesia and why?

5.3 Why might a patient having a spinal anaesthetic for surgery become hypotensive and bradycardic? How would you treat this?

5.4 What symptoms and signs in a patient would suggest local anaesthetic toxicity? How would you treat this?

True/false questions

5.1 Regional anaesthesia:
  a offers no advantage to patients with chronic respiratory disease;
  b may increase blood loss during surgery;
  c causes less disturbance of concurrent disease requiring medical therapy;
  d may hinder access for the surgeon during a laparotomy.

5.2 Local anaesthetic drugs can be used:
  a intra-arterially after the application of a tourniquet;
  b by direct injection into nerves;
  c subcutaneously;
  d intrathecally.

5.3 When performing epidural anaesthesia:
  a the needle must be inserted below the second lumbar vertebra (L2);
  b the correct position of the needle is identified by the appearance of CSF;
  c the volume of local anaesthetic drug injected has no effect on the extent of anaesthesia;
  d a combination of local anaesthetic and opioid can be used.

5.4 Contraindication to performing spinal anaesthesia include:
  a coagulopathy;
  b severe aortic stenosis;
  c local skin sepsis;
  d major trauma.

5.5 Local anaesthetic toxicity:
  a may be caused despite using a safe dose of the drug;
  b may initially present with grand mal convulsions;
  c should initially be managed by raising the patient's legs to treat hypotension;
  d is an uncommon complication of epidural anaesthesia.

6

Special circumstances

The principles underlying any anaesthetic have been covered in earlier chapters. However, there are a number of anaesthetic subspecialties where there are significant differences in practice and they merit a brief introduction. In addition, there are some anaesthetic-related complications that, although rare, need to be considered in any understanding of the specialty.

Anaesthesia for emergency surgery

It is assumed that patients who need anaesthetising for emergency surgery will not have an empty stomach, which poses an increased risk of regurgitation and aspiration into the lungs of acidic stomach contents. The greatest risk is during induction of anaesthesia but some patients are also at risk during extubation and recovery. The incidence of complications appears to be related to both the volume ($>25\,\text{mL}$) and pH (<2.5) of the material aspirated. Factors predisposing to aspiration include:

- *A full stomach.* An inadequate period of starvation (emergency patients), increased gastrointestinal contents secondary to bowel obstruction, distension following face-mask ventilation.
- *Delayed gastric emptying.* Drugs (especially opiates), trauma (particularly head injury), peritoneal irritation, blood in the stomach, pain and anxiety.
- *Obstetric patients (see below).*
- *Other causes.* A history of gastro-oesophageal reflux, hiatus hernia, obesity, head-down position, presence of a bulbar palsy, oesophageal pouch or stricture.

Consequently, in these patients measures will be taken to prevent aspiration and the majority will be intubated in order to secure and protect their airway. In order to achieve this as safely as possible, the technique used for induction of anaesthesia is slightly modified and referred to as rapid-sequence induction or RSI.

Reducing the risks of aspiration

A variety of methods are used, alone or in combination.

1 Reduction of residual gastric volume:
   - an adequate period of preoperative starvation;
   - avoidance of drugs that delay gastric emptying;
   - insertion of a nasogastric tube and aspiration of gastric contents;

Clinical Anaesthesia Lecture Notes, Fourth Edition. Carl Gwinnutt and Matthew Gwinnutt.
© 2012 John Wiley & Sons, Ltd. Published 2012 by John Wiley & Sons, Ltd.

○ use of pro-kinetic drugs, such as metoclopramide.
2 Increase pH of gastric contents:
  ○ sodium citrate to neutralize gastric acid;
  ○ H_2 antagonists, such as ranitidine;
  ○ proton pump inhibitors, for example omeprazole, lansoprazole (conveniently available in an oro-dispersible preparation).
3 Use of cricoid pressure (see below).

Cricoid pressure (Sellick's manoeuvre)

Aspiration of regurgitated gastric contents is a life-threatening complication of anaesthesia and every effort must be made to minimize the risk. Cricoid pressure is used as a physical barrier to regurgitation in patients at high risk of regurgitation. The cricoid cartilage is the only complete ring of cartilage in the larynx. Pressure applied to its anterior aspect forces the whole ring posteriorly, compressing the oesophagus against the body of the sixth cervical vertebra, occluding it and preventing regurgitation. The manoeuvre is carried out by an assistant, applying pressure as the patient loses consciousness using the thumb and index finger of their right hand whilst the other hand stabilizes the patient's neck from behind (Fig. 6.1). Cricoid pressure should be maintained even if the patient starts to actively vomit, as the risk of aspiration is greater than the theoretical risk of oesophageal rupture.

Rapid sequence induction of anaesthesia

Preoxygenation is achieved as already described, during which time monitors are attached, venous access is secured if not already done and an IV infusion started. Suction apparatus is switched on and a rigid Yankeur sucker attached and placed within immediate reach of the anaesthetist. A check is made that the anaesthetic assistant is able to apply cricoid pressure effectively and they understand it is not to be released until instruction is given by the anaesthetist to do so. Patients must also be warned that they will feel gentle pressure on their neck.

When preoxygenation is judged to be adequate, gentle cricoid pressure (10 N) is applied and the predetermined dose of the induction drug is given into a fast-running IV infusion and, as consciousness is lost, the cricoid pressure is increased

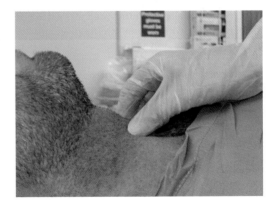

Figure 6.1 Cricoid pressure (Sellick's manoeuvre).

(30 N). The dose of suxamethonium is given and the facemask is held against the patient's face, but manual ventilation is not performed. To do so would risk forcing oxygen into the stomach, distending it and increasing the risk of regurgitation. The patient is observed for the fasciculations caused by suxamethonium and once they have stopped, direct laryngoscopy is performed and the patient intubated. The cuff of the tracheal tube is inflated and satisfactory position of the tube confirmed as already described. When the anaesthetist is confident that the tube is in the trachea, cricoid pressure is released.

Anaesthesia and surgery then continue as described previously, using either an inhalational or intravenous technique to maintain anaesthesia. A non-depolarizing neuromuscular blocking drug is given when there is evidence, either clinically or by using a nerve stimulator, that the effect of suxamethonium is diminishing. It is common to pass a nasogastric (or orogastric) tube during anaesthesia to allow aspiration of gastric contents. However, this does not always guarantee complete emptying of the stomach. Therefore at the end of surgery, patients are extubated once there is evidence of return of their laryngeal reflexes (for example, coughing), with them sat up at 30° or, if this is not appropriate, on their side.

Anaesthesia for obstetric patients

Obstetric patients may require anaesthesia for a variety of surgical procedures but the commonest is for a caesarean section, either electively or as an emergency, usually when the mother is already in labour. The following is an outline of the principles of anaesthesia. It is important to note that, whichever technique is used, adequate prophylaxis against acid aspiration is mandatory:

- elective caesarean section – an H2 antagonist or proton pump inhibitor the night before and morning of surgery;
- emergency caesarean section – an H2 antagonist and 30 ml 0.3 M sodium citrate immediately before going to theatre.

There are two main anaesthetic techniques for a caesarean section: regional (epidural or spinal anaesthesia) and general anaesthesia. Current recommendations are that caesarean section should wherever possible be performed under regional anaesthesia as this is associated with lower maternal and foetal mortality.

Regional anaesthesia is now the choice for almost all elective (90%) and most emergency caesarean sections, and the majority of these are spinal anaesthetics as this provides rapid, reliable and intense anaesthesia. It is recommended that women are offered intrathecal diamorphine as part of the technique, as this improves postoperative pain control and reduces the need for further analgesia.

The principles of spinal anaesthesia are as described in Chapter 5. Most anaesthetists perform the spinal with the patient sitting as this makes the midline easier to identify and is associated with slightly faster onset of block. The main problems associated with this technique are that unlike general and epidural anaesthesia, it is time limited and hypotension is more common. The latter is usually managed with a combination of an IV fluid preload and an infusion of phenylephrine (30–60 µg/min).

Epidurals are predominantly used to provide analgesia during labour. The extent and intensity of the block can be increased (anaesthesia) to allow caesarean section to take place. However, this is a relatively slow process and there is a risk of inadequate anaesthesia due to inadequate or absent block of some nerve roots. The technique and other problems are as described in Chapter 5.

The commonest reasons for the use of general anaesthesia are the urgency of the caesarean section (usually because of an immediate threat to the life of the mother or foetus), refusal of a regional technique by the patient, failure or contraindication of the regional technique. There are a number of problems specifically associated with general anaesthesia:

- There is an increased risk of regurgitation and aspiration. This is due to the progesterone-induced relaxation of the lower oesophageal sphincter and increased intra-abdominal pressure from the presence of the gravid uterus. This is exacerbated by the fact that in labour, gastric emptying is very slow. All pregnant women requiring general anaesthesia are regarded as having a full stomach and receive antacid prophylaxis as described above and anaesthesia is induced using an RSI with cricoid pressure. During emergency surgery, a gastric tube is passed to try and empty the stomach, and patients should be extubated once there is evidence of return of their laryngeal reflexes (e.g. coughing) and sat up at 30°.
- Failed intubation is more common in obstetric patients (1:300 compared to 1:3000 non-obstetric patients). This is primarily due to anatomical factors, in particular enlargement of breast tissue, engorgement of the airway mucosa and the fact that most women have a full set of teeth. When combined with the fact that the FRC is reduced and oxygen consumption increased, the pregnant woman will desaturate and become hypoxic remarkably quickly during repeated attempts at intubation. Attention must be paid to ensuring full preoxygenation, head and neck position must be optimized, and intubation must only be attempted at the point of maximal action of suxamethonium. If intubation fails, institute a failed intubation drill. Oxygenation is more important than intubation.
- Maternal awareness as a result of the use of inadequate doses of the induction and inhalational drugs in an attempt to avoid oversedating the baby. Adequate doses of drugs must be given; 'flat' babies can be resuscitated by a paediatrician.

Aortocaval compression

As the gravid uterus enlarges through the pregnancy, it compresses the inferior vena cava, reducing venous return to the heart and therefore cardiac output and blood pressure. The effect is maximal by 36 weeks gestation, worse in the supine position and exacerbated by the sympathetic block produced by epidurals and spinals. In addition, compression of the aorta may occur, reducing blood pressure and flow in the uterine arteries that may cause foetal hypoxia. Both of these effects can be prevented by using a 15° left lateral tilt in the supine patient and it is essential that, whichever technique of anaesthesia is used for a caesarean section, the mother is placed in this position.

Anaesthesia for thoracotomy

Surgery to the chest contents or to the anterior thoracic spine via a thoracotomy poses significant challenges for the anaesthetist – in particular the need to isolate and ventilate both lungs independently. This allows one lung to be deflated whilst ventilation is maintained via the other. The indications for this are to:

- facilitate surgical access, for example to the oesophagus, thoracic spine, the deflated lung;
- avoid contamination from one lung to the other, for example infection, bleeding;
- allow differential ventilation of both lungs, for example in the presence of a large leak due to a bulla.

The most popular method of achieving one-lung ventilation (OLV) is by the insertion of a double-lumen tube (Fig. 6.2). A variety of suitable tubes are available, either made out of natural

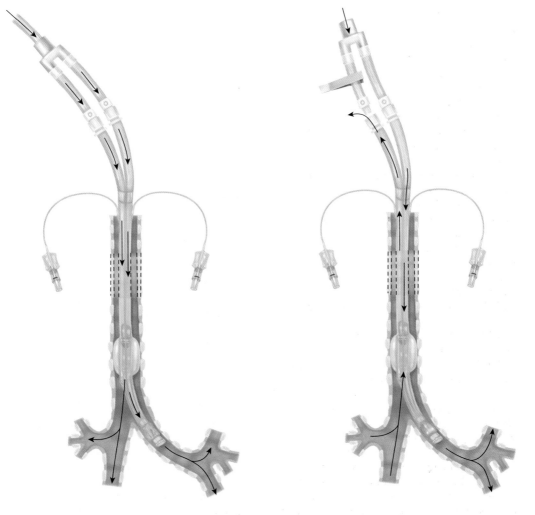

Figure 6.2 (a) Left sided double lumen tube, bilateral ventilation. (b) Left sided double lumen tube, ventilation of left lung only.

'red' rubber or PVC (single use). The principle of these tubes is that one lumen is longer and designed to be introduced specifically into the left or right main bronchus (hence they are referred to as left- or right-sided endobronchial tubes). A small cuff on this bronchial lumen provides a gas-tight seal and allows ventilation of the lung on this side. The other, shorter lumen ends proximal to the carina, has a larger cuff and gas delivered down this lumen predominantly enters the non-intubated bronchus. These tubes are considerably larger than standard tracheal tubes and can be difficult to insert to lie in the correct position. Therefore after insertion, their position is checked clinically by checking that both lungs can be ventilated independently, and many anaesthetists will confirm placement by inserting a bronchoscope.

After insertion, both lungs are usually ventilated (Fig. 6.2a). At the point that one lung needs to be deflated, the cuff on the endobronchial lumen is inflated and ventilation continued into this lung. The proximal end of the shorter lumen is disconnected and ventilation via this lumen is stopped (the tube from the ventilator, proximal to the disconnection must be clamped). The gas in the lung can then escape and the lung collapses (Fig. 6.2b).

A left-sided tube is usually chosen as this is slightly easier to insert into the correct position and less likely to obstruct a lobar bronchus. Right-sided tubes are usually reserved for operations involving the left main bronchus.

One of the main problems of OLV is that it creates a shunt, as blood from the right ventricle is now passing through non-ventilated lung and therefore does not become oxygenated before returning to the systemic circulation, resulting in significant hypoxia. In normal lungs, collapse of the lung reduces the blood flow through it and reduces the magnitude of the shunt. All that may be required to maintain a normal SpO_2 is an increase in the inspired oxygen concentration. If this fails, or the patient has significant underlying pulmonary disease, there are three options:

- partial reinflation of the collapsed lung and the application of a small amount of continuous positive airway pressure (CPAP) to the lumen with 100% oxygen;
- intermittent reinflation of the lung with 100% oxygen;
- return to two lung ventilation and use surgical retraction of the lung.

At the end of the surgical procedure a chest drain is usually inserted to allow drainage of any blood or fluid from the pleural cavity and prevent the formation of a pneumothorax from any gas leak from the lung surface. Finally, the deflated lung must be reinflated. This is usually done by reconnecting the ventilator circuit and ventilating the lungs manually at slightly increased peak inflation pressure to fully re-expand the whole lung.

Aspiration of gastric contents

Despite a seemingly appropriate preoperative fasting period, or despite taking all of the precautions outlined above for patients identified as at risk, occasionally regurgitation and aspiration still occur. Signs suggesting aspiration include:

- coughing during induction or recovery from anaesthesia, or during anaesthesia using a supra-glottic airway device;
- gastric contents in the pharynx at laryngoscopy, or around the edge of the facemask;
- if severe, progressive hypoxia, bronchospasm and respiratory obstruction.

Occasionally, aspiration may go completely unnoticed during anaesthesia, with the development of hypoxia, hypotension and respiratory failure postoperatively.

Management

Aspiration at induction

- Maintain a patent airway and place the patient head-down and on his or her side, preferably the left; intubation is relatively easier on this side.
- Aspirate any material from the pharynx, preferably under direct vision (use a laryngoscope).

(i) Neuromuscular blocking drugs not given; surgery not urgent:

- Give 100% oxygen via a facemask.
- Allow the patient to recover, give oxygen to maintain a satisfactory SpO_2.
- Treat bronchospasm with salbutamol or ipratroprium as described in Chapter 8.

- Take a chest X-ray and organize regular physiotherapy.
- Depending on degree of aspiration, consider monitoring on the ITU or HDU.

(ii) Neuromuscular blocking drugs not given; surgery essential:

- Get help, empty the stomach with a nasogastric tube and instil 30 mL sodium citrate.
- After allowing the patient to recover, continue using either a regional technique or a rapid-sequence induction and intubation.
- After intubation, aspirate the tracheobronchial tree and consider bronchoscopy.
- Treat bronchospasm as above.
- Postoperatively, arrange for a chest X-ray and physiotherapy.
- Recover in the ITU or HDU with oxygen therapy.
- Postoperative ventilation may be required.

(iii) Neuromuscular blocking drugs given:

- Intubate with a cuffed tracheal tube to secure the airway.
- Aspirate the tracheobronchial tree before starting positive pressure ventilation.
- Consider bronchopulmonary lavage with saline.
- Treat bronchospasm as above.
- Pass a nasogastric tube and empty the stomach.
- If the patient is stable (not hypoxic or hypotensive), surgery can be continued with postoperative care as described above.

If oxygen saturation remains low despite 100% oxygen, consider the possibility of obstruction and the need for fibre optic bronchoscopy.

Aspiration intraoperatively with supra-glottic airway

- Get help.
- Stop surgery if safe to do so.
- Turn patient into left lateral position with head down tilt.
- Remove supra-glottic airway device and suction oro-pharynx.
- Maintain ventilation with 100% oxygen, ensure ongoing anaesthesia.
- Trained assistant to apply cricoid pressure.
- Give a fast-acting neuromuscular-blocking drug and intubate the trachea.

If aspiration is suspected in a patient postoperatively, treat as for (i) above. There is no place for routine administration of large-dose steroids. Antibiotics should be given according to local protocols. In those patients with bronchospasm resistant to treatment, or with persistent hypoxia or hypotension, surgery should be deferred unless it is potentially lifesaving. Instead they should be transferred to the ITU for ventilation, with additional, invasive cardiorespiratory monitoring as needed.

Anaphylaxis

Most adverse drug reactions in anaesthesia are mild and transient, consisting mainly of localized urticaria as a result of cutaneous histamine release. The incidence of anaphylaxis caused by anaesthetic drugs is between 1:10 000 and 1:20 000 drug administrations, and is more common in females. Of those reported to the Medicines Control Agency, 10% involved a fatality compared to 3.7% for drugs overall. This probably reflects the frequency with which anaesthetic drugs are given intravenously. Clinical features include (in order of frequency):

- severe hypotension;
- severe bronchospasm;
- widespread flushing;
- hypoxaemia;
- urticaria;
- angioedema, which may involve the airway;
- pruritus, nausea and vomiting.

Cardiovascular collapse is the most common and severe feature. Asthmatics often develop bronchospasm that is resistant to treatment and any circumstance that reduces the patient's catecholamine response (such as beta blockers, spinal anaesthesia) will increase the severity.

Anaphylaxis involves the degranulation of mast cells and basophils, either as a result of an allergic (IgE mediated) or non-allergic (non-IgE mediated) reaction, liberating histamine, 5-hydroxytryptamine (5-HT) and associated vasoactive substances. The latter used to be called an anaphylactoid reaction, but this term is no longer used. The European Academy of Allergology and Clinical Immunology Nomenclature Committee have proposed the following broad definition:

> Anaphylaxis is a severe, life-threatening generalized or systemic hypersensitivity reaction.

Causes of allergic reactions

- *Anaesthetic drugs*:
  - muscle relaxants (>50%): suxamethonium, rocuronium, atracurium, vecuronium;
  - induction agents (5%): thiopentone, propofol.
- *Latex* (17%).
- *Antibiotics* (8%):
  - penicillin (<1% of patients may cross-react to modern cephalosporins).
- *Intravenous fluids*:
  - colloids (3%); haemaccel, gelofusin.
- *Opioids* (2%).

Immediate management

The following advice is based on guidelines issued by the Resuscitation Council (UK) and AAGBI (see useful information section):

- Discontinue all drugs likely to have triggered the reaction.
- Call for help.
- Maintain a patent airway, administer 100% oxygen, elevate the patient's legs providing ventilation is not compromised.
- Give adrenaline, 50 µg *slowly* intravenously (0.5 mL of 1:10 000) under ECG control. A dilution of 1:100 000 adrenaline (10 µg/mL) allows better titration and reduces the risk of adverse effects. If no ECG available, give 0.5 mg intramuscularly (0.5 mL of 1:1000). If there is no improvement within 5 min, give a further dose.
- Give high flow oxygen, 10–15 L/min.
- Ensure adequate ventilation:
  - intubation will be required if spontaneous ventilation is inadequate or in the presence of severe bronchospasm. This may be exceedingly difficult in the presence of severe laryngeal oedema. In these circumstances a needle cricothyroidotomy or surgical airway will be required.
- Support the circulation:
  - start a rapid IV infusion of fluids 10–20 mL/kg. Crystalloids initially may be safer than colloids. In the absence of a major pulse, start cardiopulmonary resuscitation using the appropriate protocol (see Chapter 8).
- Monitoring:
  - ECG, SpO_2, blood pressure, end-tidal CO_2. Establish an arterial line and check the blood gases.
  - Monitor CVP and urine output to assess adequacy of circulating volume.

Subsequent management

- *Antihistamines.* Chlorphenamine (H_1 blocker) 10–20 mg slowly IV or IM. There is no evidence for the use of H_2 blockers.
- *Steroids.* Hydrocortisone 200 mg slowly IV or IM. This helps to stop late sequelae.
- *Bronchodilators.* Salbutamol, 2.5–5.0 mg nebulized or 0.25 mg IV, ipratroprium 500 µg. Magnesium 2 g (8 mmol) slowly IV may be useful when there are severe, asthma-like features or if the patient is taking beta-blockers. Magnesium may cause flushing and may worsen hypotension.

As soon as possible these patients should be transferred to an ITU for further treatment and monitoring. Reactions vary in severity, can be biphasic, delayed in onset (particularly latex sensitivity), and prolonged. An infusion of adrenaline may be required. The possibility of a tension pneumothorax (secondary to barotrauma) causing hypotension must not be forgotten.

Investigations

The most informative is measurement of plasma mast cell tryptase levels. A blood sample should be taken immediately after treatment and repeated approximately 1 h and 6 h after the event. Elevated tryptase levels confirm that the reaction was associated with mast cell degranulation but does not distinguish between an allergic and non-allergic cause. A negative test does not completely exclude anaphylaxis. Expert advice about follow-up and identification of the cause must be arranged.

Finally, record all details in the patient's notes, and do not forget to inform the patient and the patient's general practitioner of the events, both verbally and in writing. In the UK, report adverse drug events to the Medicines and Healthcare products Regulatory Agency by completing a 'yellow card' found in the BNF.

Generalized atopy does not help predict the risk of immunologically mediated reaction to anaesthetic drugs. A previous history of 'allergy to an anaesthetic' is cause for concern and there is a high risk of cross-reactivity between drugs of the same group. These patients must be investigated appropriately.

Malignant hyperpyrexia (hyperthermia) (MH)

This is a rare inherited disorder of skeletal muscle metabolism in which there is a release of abnormally high concentrations of calcium from the sarcoplasmic reticulum causing increased muscle activity and metabolism. Excess heat production causes a rise in core temperature of at least 2 °C/h. It is triggered by exposure to the inhalational anaesthetic agents and suxamethonium. It is more common in young adults undergoing relatively minor surgery, for example for squints, hernia repair, cleft palate repair and orthopaedic surgery. The incidence is between 1:10 000 and 1:40 000 anaesthetised patients. For more detail refer to the guidance issued by the AAGBI (see useful information section).

Presentation

- A progressive rise in body temperature (this may go unnoticed unless the patient's temperature is being monitored).
- An unexplained tachycardia.
- An increased end-tidal CO_2.
- Tachypnoea in spontaneously breathing patients.
- Muscle rigidity, failure to relax after suxamethonium, especially persistent masseter spasm.
- Cardiac arrhythmias.
- A falling oxygen saturation and cyanosis.

Immediate management

- GET HELP.
- Stop all volatile anaesthetic drugs; hyperventilate with 100% oxygen.
- Maintain anaesthesia with total intravenous anaesthetic technique.
- Change the anaesthesia machine and circuits.
- Terminate surgery as soon as practical.
- Monitor core temperature.
- Give dantrolene 2–3 mg/kg IV, then 1 mg/kg boluses as required (up to 10 mg/kg may be needed).
- Start active cooling:
  - cold 0.9% saline IV;
  - expose the patient completely;
  - surface cooling – ice over axillary and femoral arteries, wet sponging and fanning to encourage cooling by evaporation;
  - consider gastric or peritoneal lavage with cold saline.
- Treat acidosis with 8.4% sodium bicarbonate 50 mmol (50 mL) IV titrated to acid-base results.
- Treat hyperkalaemia.
- Transfer the patient to the ITU as soon as possible for:
  - temperature monitoring, may be labile for up to 48 hours;
  - continuation of dantrolene to alleviate muscle rigidity;
  - monitoring of urine output for myoglobin and treatment to prevent renal failure;
  - treatment of coagulopathy.

Dantrolene

This is the only specific treatment for MH. It inhibits calcium release preventing further muscle activity. Dantrolene is orange in colour, supplied in vials containing 20 mg (plus 3 g mannitol), requires 60 mL water for reconstitution and is very slow to dissolve.

Investigation of the family

Following an episode, the patient and their family should be referred to a MH Unit for investigation of their susceptibility to MH.

Anaesthesia for malignant hyperpyrexia-susceptible patients

- Employ a regional technique using plain bupivacaine if appropriate.
- General anaesthesia:
  - use a designated vapour-free machine, new circuits and hoses;
  - TIVA using an infusion of propofol and remifentanil and oxygen-enriched air for ventilation is commonly used;
  - consider pretreatment with dantrolene (orally or IV) in those who have survived a previous episode;
  - monitor temperature, ensure cooling available.

Difficult intubation

Occasionally it is not possible to visualize the larynx, which makes it difficult or impossible to intubate the trachea. This may have been pre-dicted at the preoperative assessment or may be unexpected. A variety of techniques have been described to help solve this problem, which include the following:

- Manipulation of the thyroid cartilage (BURP manoeuvre) using **b**ackward, **u**pward, **r**ightward **p**ressure (patient's right) by an assistant to try and bring the larynx or its posterior aspect into view.
- At laryngoscopy, a 60 cm-long gum elastic bougie is inserted blindly into the trachea, over which the tracheal tube is 'railroaded' into place.
- A fibre-optic bronchoscope is introduced into the trachea via the mouth or nose, and is used as a guide over which a tube can be passed into the trachea – this technique has the advantage that it can be used in either anaesthetised or awake patients.

- An LMA or ILM can be inserted and used as a conduit to pass a tracheal tube directly or via a fibre optic bronchoscope.
- Use of indirect laryngoscopes if they are available and if you have the skills necessary to use them.

Failed intubation

Despite utilizing the techniques described above, sometimes the patient cannot be intubated. The incidence of failed intubation will depend on a number of factors including the skill and experience of the anaesthetist and the type of cases being undertaken. A failed intubation in itself is not particularly harmful, *providing oxygenation can be maintained*. Because almost all patients will have

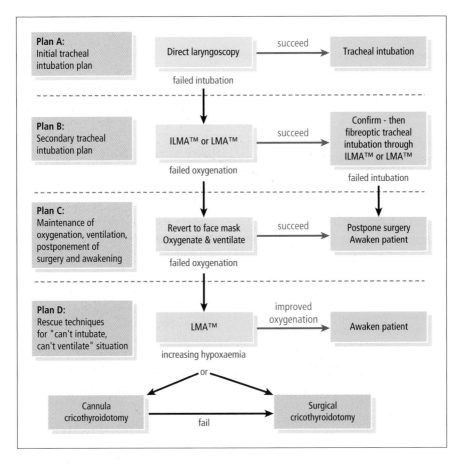

Figure 6.3 Difficult Airway Society (DAS) algorithm for managing failed tracheal intubation. Reproduced with the kind permission of the Difficult Airway Society.

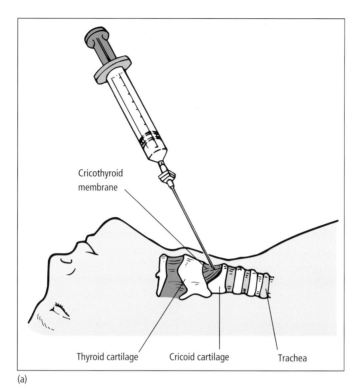

Cricothyroid
membrane

Thyroid cartilage   Cricoid cartilage   Trachea

(a)

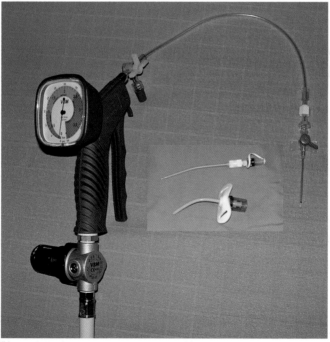

(b)

Figure 6.4 (a) Needle cricothyroidotomy. (b) Oxygen delivery system (Manujet) attached to an IV cannula. The pressure of oxygen delivered is controlled by the lower black knob and displayed on the dial. Oxygen is delivered by squeezing the vertical trigger. Inset: purpose-made cannula and stylet for cricothyroid puncture.

been given neuromuscular blocking drugs they will be dependent on the anaesthetist for this. Consequently, prior to every intubation, 'back-up plans' are needed to allow the safe implementation of different techniques of intubation, whilst ensuring that the patient does not come to harm from hypoxia. Such plans will need to take into account the likelihood of any difficulty (as anticipated at the preoperative assessment), risk of aspiration and urgency of surgery, and are often referred to as plans A, B, C and D. Such a system has been developed by the Difficult Airway Society (DAS) and is outlined in Fig. 6.3. Further details are available on the DAS website (see useful information section).

> In every circumstance where difficulty is encountered with tracheal intubation, summon help immediately.

Plan A – the initial plan to use direct laryngoscopy to intubate the trachea. If this fails . . .

Plan B – the secondary intubation plan. A supraglottic airway is used to secure the airway and ventilate the patient. If oxygenation can be maintained, it can then be used as a conduit to attempt intubation. If intubation fails and is essential for surgery or oxygenation cannot be maintained . . .

Plan C – remove the supraglottic airway and use a facemask to oxygenate the patient. If this is successful, depending on the urgency of surgery, wake the patient up. If this fails . . .

Plan D – insert a different size/type of supraglottic airway. If oxygenation is successful, wake the patient up. If it fails, use a rescue technique, cannula or surgical cricothyroidotomy, to oxygenate the patient.

Any patient whose airway has been traumatized, either as a result of repeated attempts at intubation or following surgical intervention, is at risk of developing oedema and airway obstruction at extubation. These patients should be admitted to an appropriate critical care area postoperatively and may require endoscopy prior to extubation.

Full details of the difficulties encountered and any solutions must be documented in the patient's notes. The patient must be given verbal and written details (consider 'MedicAlert' type device) and details sent to his or her GP. The DAS has developed an 'Airway Alert' form that contains a summary of airway management and contacts for further details (see useful information section).

Needle cricothyroidotomy

This technique is used only *when all others have failed to maintain oxygenation*. The cricothyroid membrane is identified and punctured using a large bore cannula (12–14 g) attached to a syringe. Aspiration of air confirms that the tip of the cannula lies within the trachea. The cannula is then angled to about 45° caudally and advanced off the needle into the trachea (Fig. 6.4a). In order to overcome the high resistance of the narrow cannula lumen the oxygen delivered must be from a high pressure supply (Fig. 6.4b). While holding the cannula in place, oxygen is insufflated for 1 s, followed by a 4 s rest. Expiration occurs via the upper airway as normal along with the escape of excess gas during insufflation. This technique adequately oxygenates the patient but only results in minimal carbon dioxide elimination, and is therefore limited to about 30 min use while help is obtained and a definitive airway is created. Extreme care must be taken if this technique is used in the presence of upper airway obstruction. Progressively more oxygen is delivered to the lungs by the high pressure source that cannot escape, eventually causing a pneumothorax. Increasingly, specifically developed kits are used should the need arise (see useful information section). These contain a cannula that connects directly via a standard 15 mm connector to a breathing circuit, along with everything needed for its insertion. The diameter of the cannula allows adequate volumes to ensure oxygenation and ventilation (see useful information section).

📖 FURTHER USEFUL INFORMATION

www.aagbi.org/sites/default/files/anaphylaxis _2009_0.pdf

[The Association of Anaesthetists of Great Britain & Ireland. Suspected anaphylactic reactions associated with anaesthesia. Revised 2009.]

http://www.aagbi.org/sites/default/files/MH% 20guideline%20for%20web.pdf

[The Association of Anaesthetists of Great Britain & Ireland guidelines for treatment of malignant hyperthermia.2007.]

http://ceaccp.oxfordjournals.org/content/8/5/ 157.full.pdf+html

[Review of large-bore cricothyroidotomy devices.]

http://www.das.uk.com/

[The Difficult Airway Society website contains guidance on management of airway emergencies, including failed intubation drills.]

http://nice.org.uk/CG132

[NICE guidelines for the management of patients undergoing caesarean section, including anaesthetic recommendations]

www.oaa-anaes.ac.uk/

[The Obstetric Anaesthetists' Association website.]

www.resus.org.uk/pages/reaction.pdf

[Resuscitation Council UK. Emergency Treatment of Anaphylactic Reactions. Guidelines for healthcare providers. Revised January 2008.]

www.thoracic-anesthesia.com

[American site, lots of references and great bronchoscopy simulator.]

All websites last accessed February 2012.

? SELF-ASSESSMENT

Short-answer questions

6.1 What factors predispose to regurgitation and aspiration of gastric contents? How can the risks be reduced?

6.2 What are the clinical signs that would suggest a patient is having an anaphylactic reaction? What would be your immediate management?

6.3 What are the clinical signs that would suggest a patient is developing malignant hyperthermia? What would be your immediate and long-term management?

6.4 Describe the immediate management of an elective surgical patient who cannot be intubated.

True/false questions

6.1 Cricoid pressure:

a is used to prevent vomiting during induction of anaesthesia;

b works by compressing the oesophagus between the cricoid cartilage and the vertebral column;

c should start before the patient is anaesthetised;

d can be released as soon as the tracheal tube is inserted.

6.2 When anaesthetising a patient for a caesarean section:

a general anaesthesia is the technique of choice;

b pregnancy at term is a risk factor for aspiration on induction;

c spinal anaesthesia is often associated with significant hypotension needing vasopressors;

d the operating table should be kept level to avoid the risk of the patient falling off.

6.3 One-lung ventilation:

a is performed to allow improved surgical access;

b is most often achieved by using a specially designed double-lumen tracheal tube;

c using a left-sided tube is more likely to obstruct a lobar bronchus;

d results in significant V/Q mismatch during anaesthesia.

6.4 In the management of anaphylaxis:

a IV hydrocortisone is the single most important treatment;

b the dose of adrenaline is 0.5 mL of 1 in 10 000 IM;

c intubation may be difficult due to jaw rigidity;

d the patient will need monitoring in a critical care unit after the initial treatment.

6.5 In the management of malignant hyperthermia (MH):

a anaesthesia should be maintained with a propofol infusion;

b surgery must be stopped immediately;

c verapamil is the treatment of choice;

d the patient should be monitored for AKI secondary to rhabdomyolysis.

7

Post-anaesthesia care

The vast majority of patients recover from anaesthesia and surgery uneventfully but a small and unpredictable number suffer complications. It is now accepted that all patients should be nursed by trained staff, in an area with appropriate facilities to deal with any of the problems that may arise while recovering from anaesthesia. Such specialized areas are referred to as the post-anaesthesia care unit (PACU) or recovery unit. Most patients will be nursed on a trolley capable of being tipped head-down. Patients who have undergone prolonged surgery or where a prolonged stay in PACU is expected, may be nursed on their beds to minimize the number of transfers. Some patients, who have undergone specialist surgery – for example cardiac surgery patients – may be taken directly to a critical care area.

The post-anaesthesia care unit

Each patient in the PACU should be cared for in an area equipped with:

- oxygen supply plus appropriate circuits for giving it;
- suction;
- ECG monitoring;
- pulse oximeter;
- non-invasive blood pressure monitor.

In addition the following must be available immediately:

- *Airway equipment.* Oral and nasal airways, a range of tracheal tubes, laryngoscopes, a bronchoscope and the instruments to perform a cricothyroidotomy and tracheostomy.
- *Breathing and ventilation equipment.* Self-inflating bag-valve-masks, a mechanical ventilator and a chest drain set.
- *Circulation equipment.* A defibrillator, drugs for CPR, a range of IV solutions, pressure infusers and devices for IV access.
- *Drugs.* For resuscitation and anaesthesia. Many areas also store dantrolene for treating malignant hyperthermia (see Chapter 6) and lipid emulsion for treatment of local anaesthetic toxicity (see Chapter 5).
- *Monitoring equipment.* Transducers and a monitor capable of displaying two or three pressure waveforms, an end-tidal carbon dioxide

Clinical Anaesthesia Lecture Notes, Fourth Edition. Carl Gwinnutt and Matthew Gwinnutt.
© 2012 John Wiley & Sons, Ltd. Published 2012 by John Wiley & Sons, Ltd.

monitor, and a thermometer. This may be needed in patients who have undergone complex surgery with invasive monitoring that is continued in the immediate postoperative period or occasionally those who require resuscitation.

Discharge of the patient

The anaesthetist's responsibility to the patient does not end with termination of the anaesthetic. Although care is handed over to the PACU staff (nurse or equivalent), the responsibility ultimately remains with the anaesthetist until the patient is discharged from the PACU. If there are inadequate numbers of PACU staff to care for a newly admitted patient, the anaesthetist should adopt this role.

> A patient who cannot maintain his/her own airway should never be left alone.

The length of time any patient spends in PACU will depend upon a variety of factors, including duration and type of surgery, anaesthetic technique, and the occurrence of any complications. Most units have a policy determining the minimum length of stay (usually around 30 min), and agreed discharge criteria (Table 7.1).

Table 7.1 Minimum criteria for discharge from PACU

- Fully conscious and able to maintain own airway (although patient may still be 'sleepy')
- Adequate breathing
- Stable cardiovascular system, with minimal bleeding from the surgical site
- Adequate pain relief
- Warm

Postoperative complications and their management

Hypoxaemia

This is the most important respiratory complication after anaesthesia and surgery. It may start at recovery and in some patients persist for 3 days or more after surgery. The presence of cyanosis is very insensitive and, when detectable, means the arterial PO_2 will be <8 kPa (55 mmHg), corresponding to a haemoglobin saturation of 85%. The advent of pulse oximetry has had a major impact on the prevention of hypoxaemia and should be used routinely in all patients. If hypoxaemia is severe, persistent, or when there is any doubt, arterial blood gas analysis should be performed. Hypoxaemia can be caused by a number of factors, either alone or in combination:

- alveolar hypoventilation;
- ventilation and perfusion mismatch within the lungs;
- diffusion hypoxia;
- pulmonary diffusion defects;
- a reduced inspired oxygen concentration.

Alveolar hypoventilation

This is the commonest cause of hypoxaemia after general anaesthesia. It is caused by a degree of respiratory depression leading to an insufficient flow of oxygen into the alveoli to replace that taken up by the blood. As a result alveolar PO_2 (PAO_2) and arterial PO_2 (PaO_2) fall. In most patients, increasing their inspired oxygen concentration will restore both. This is the rationale for giving all patients who have had a general anaesthetic oxygen therapy. Fig. 7.1 shows the variation of PaO_2 with ventilation (minute volume). Note the effect of giving 30% oxygen to a patient whose ventilation is 2 L/min (normally 5 L/min): The PaO_2 rises from being barely adequate to supranormal. This is because 30% oxygen contains nearly one-and-a-half times the amount of oxygen that is in air. If ventilation is further reduced, a point is eventually reached where there is only ventilation of the anatomical 'dead space' – that is, the volume of the airways that plays no part in gas exchange. If this occurs, irrespective of the inspired oxygen concentration, no oxygen reaches the alveoli and profound hypoxaemia will follow. Note that an increase in minute volume above normal only increases oxygenation minimally. This is because it does not alter the main determinant of alveolar oxygen tension, the inspired PO_2. Hypoventilation is always accompanied by hypercapnia, as there is an inverse relationship between alveolar ventilation and arterial carbon dioxide ($PaCO_2$) (Fig. 7.2).

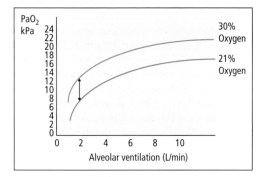

Figure 7.1 Graph showing the relationship between PaO_2 and alveolar ventilation at two different inspired oxygen concentrations.

Common causes of hypoventilation include:

- *Obstruction of the airway.* Most often secondary to a reduced level of consciousness but also may be due to vomit, blood, or swelling (for example, post-thyroid surgery). Partial obstruction causes noisy breathing; in complete obstruction there is little noise despite vigorous efforts. There may be a characteristic 'see-saw' or paradoxical pattern of ventilation. A tracheal tug may be seen. The risk of obstruction can be reduced by recovering patients in the lateral position, particularly those recovering from surgery where there is a risk of bleeding into the airway (as in ear, nose and throat (ENT) surgery), or regurgitation (bowel obstruction or a history of reflux). If it is not possible to turn the patient (for instance, after a hip replacement),

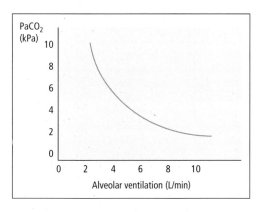

Figure 7.2 Graph showing the relationship between $PaCO_2$ and alveolar ventilation.

perform a chin lift or jaw thrust (see Chapter 4). An oropharyngeal or nasopharyngeal airway may be required to help maintain the airway (see Chapter 4). As the patient begins to obey commands they can be sat up at 30° if it is safe to do so.

> No patient should be handed to the care of the PACU staff with noisy respiration of unknown cause.

- *Central respiratory depression.* This is usually due to drugs given during anaesthesia. Both anaesthetic drugs and opioid analgesics depress the normal increase in ventilation seen in response to hypoxia and hypercarbia, and the residual effects of these drugs are commonly present in the recovery period. If ventilation is inadequate it may need to be supported until the effects of the drugs have worn off, or, in the case of severe opioid-induced respiratory depression, the specific antagonist naloxone may be given (see Chapter 3).
- *Impaired mechanics of ventilation.* Pain, particularly after upper abdominal or thoracic surgery, prevents coughing, leading to sputum retention and atelectasis. The solution to this is provision of adequate analgesia (consider central neural block). Residual neuromuscular blockade causes weakness and impaired ventilation. The patient will usually show signs of unsustained, jerky movements with rapid, shallow breathing, hypertension and tachycardia. The diagnosis may be confirmed by using a peripheral nerve stimulator, which may show evidence of fade with a tetanic stimulus (see Chapter 2). The patient should be given oxygen, reassured, sat upright to improve the efficiency of ventilation, and a (further) dose of neostigmine and an anticholinergic given. If rocuronium has been given, sugammadex may be used.
- *Diaphragmatic splinting.* Abdominal distension and obesity cause the diaphragm to be pushed into the thorax and increase the work of breathing. Sitting these patients up helps them greatly.
- *Cerebral haemorrhage or ischaemia.* May cause direct damage to the respiratory centre or, more commonly, a deeply unconscious patient unable to maintain a patent airway.

- *Pneumothorax or haemothorax.* Both will prevent ventilation of the underlying lung and will require the insertion of a chest drain.
- *Hypothermia.* Reduces ventilation but, in the absence of any contributing factors, it is usually adequate for the body's needs.

Ventilation and perfusion mismatch within the lungs

Normally, alveolar ventilation (V) and perfusion with blood (Q) are well matched (V/Q = 1) and the haemoglobin in blood leaving the lungs is almost fully saturated with oxygen (97–98%). This is disturbed (ventilation/perfusion (V/Q) mismatch) during anaesthesia and the recovery period, with development of areas where:

- *Perfusion exceeds ventilation (V/Q < 1).* This results in blood with reduced oxygen content.
- *Ventilation exceeds perfusion (V/Q > 1).* This can be considered wasted ventilation. Only a small additional volume of oxygen is taken up as the haemoglobin is already almost fully saturated.

In the most extreme situation, there is perfusion of areas of the lung but no ventilation (V/Q = 0). Blood leaving these areas remains 'venous' and is often referred to as 'shunted blood' (that is, it is effectively shunted directly from the venous to arterial system). This is then mixed with oxygenated blood leaving ventilated areas of the lungs. The net result is:

- Blood perfusing alveoli ventilated with air has an oxygen content of approximately 20 mL/100 mL of blood.
- Blood perfusing unventilated alveoli remains venous, with an oxygen content of 15 mL/100 mL of blood.
- The final oxygen content of blood leaving the lungs will be dependent on the relative proportions of shunted blood and non-shunted blood.

> For an equivalent blood flow, areas of V/Q < 1 decrease oxygen content more than areas of V/Q > 1 can increase it, even if the inspired oxygen concentration is increased to 100%.

The aetiology of V/Q mismatch is multifactorial but the following are recognized as being of importance:

- Mechanical ventilation reduces cardiac output. This reduces perfusion of non-dependent areas of the lungs, whilst maintaining ventilation. This is worst in the lateral position, when the upper lung is better ventilated and the lower lung better perfused.
- A reduced functional residual capacity (FRC). In supine, anaesthetised patients, particularly those over 50 years of age, the FRC falls below their closing capacity – the lung volume below which some airways close and distal alveoli are no longer ventilated. Eventually, areas of atelectasis develop, mainly in dependent areas of the lung, as a result of perfusion but no ventilation.
- Pain restricts breathing and coughing, leading to poor ventilation of the lung bases, sputum retention, basal atelectasis and, ultimately, infection. The highest incidence of this is seen in the following circumstances:
  ○ smokers;
  ○ obesity;
  ○ pre-existing lung disease;
  ○ elderly;
  ○ after upper gastrointestinal or thoracic surgery;
  ○ three days after surgery.

The effects of small areas of V/Q mismatch can be compensated for by increasing the inspired oxygen concentration. However, because of the disproportionate effect of areas where V/Q < 1, once more than 30% of the pulmonary blood flow is passing through such areas, even breathing 100% oxygen will not eliminate hypoxaemia. The oxygen content of the blood leaving alveoli ventilated with 100% oxygen will only have increased by 1 mL/100 mL of blood over what was achieved when being ventilated with air (Table 7.2). This is insufficient to offset the lack from the areas of low V/Q. Oxygen therapy is relatively ineffective when the cause of hypoxaemia is V/Q mismatch compared to when hypoventilation exists. Treatment should be aimed at optimizing ventilation of non aerated alveoli. The simplest manoeuvre is to sit the patient upright in bed, which relieves upward pressure on the diaphragm, easing the work of breathing and so improving aeration of the lung bases. The next manoeuvre is to apply continuous positive airways pressure (CPAP) via a closely fitting face mask and a suitable circuit. This recruits alveoli but may be poorly tolerated by patients for periods of more than a few hours.

Table 7.2 Effect of alveolar oxygen concentration on oxygen content of blood

	Alveolar oxygen concentration (%)	Haemoglobin saturation (%)	Oxygen content (mL/100 mL blood)
Alveoli containing air	21	97	20
Alveoli containing oxygen	100	100	21
Non-ventilated alveoli	Very low	75	15

> Oxygen therapy is relatively ineffective at relieving hypoxaemia where the cause is V/Q mismatch compared to hypoventilation. Opening (recruiting) unventilated alveoli is likely to be more effective.

Diffusion hypoxia

Nitrous oxide absorbed during anaesthesia has to be excreted during recovery. It is very insoluble in blood, and so rapidly diffuses down a concentration gradient into the alveoli, where it reduces the partial pressure of oxygen making the patient hypoxaemic. This can be treated by giving oxygen via a facemask to increase the inspired oxygen concentration (see below).

Pulmonary diffusion defects

Any chronic condition causing thickening of the alveolar membrane, such as fibrosing alveolitis, impairs transfer of oxygen into the blood. In the recovery period it may also occur secondary to the development of pulmonary oedema following fluid overload or impaired left ventricular function. It should be treated by first administering oxygen to increase the partial pressure of oxygen in the alveoli and then by management of any underlying cause.

A reduced inspired oxygen concentration

As the inspired oxygen concentration is a prime determinant of the amount of oxygen in the alveoli, reducing this will lead to hypoxaemia. There are no circumstances where it is appropriate to administer less than 21% oxygen.

Management of hypoxaemia

All patients should be given oxygen in the immediate postoperative period to:

- counter the effects of diffusion hypoxia when nitrous oxide has been used;
- compensate for any hypoventilation;
- compensate for V/Q mismatch;
- meet the increased oxygen demand when shivering.

Patients who continue to hypoventilate, have persistent V/Q mismatch, are obese, anaemic or have ischaemic heart disease, will require additional oxygen for an extended period of time. The need for, and effectiveness of oxygen therapy is best determined either by arterial blood gas analysis or by using a pulse oximeter. Oxygen therapy should aim to maintain the SpO_2 between 94–98%, unless the patient is known to have severe COPD when a value of 88–92% is acceptable.

Devices used for delivery of oxygen

Variable-performance devices: masks or nasal cannulae

These are adequate for the majority of patients recovering from anaesthesia and surgery. The precise concentration of oxygen inspired by the patient is unknown as it is dependent upon the patient's respiratory pattern and the flow of oxygen used (usually 2–12 L/min). The inspired gas consists of a mixture of:

- oxygen flowing into the mask;
- oxygen that has accumulated under the mask during the expiratory pause;

- alveolar gas from the previous breath which has collected under the mask;
- air entrained during peak inspiratory flow from the holes in the side of the mask and from leaks between the mask and face.

The most commonly used device is the Hudson mask (Fig. 7.3a). As a guide, it will increase the inspired oxygen concentration to 25–60% with oxygen flows of 2–12 L/min.

Patients unable to tolerate a facemask who can nose breathe may find either a single foam-tipped catheter or double catheters, placed just inside the vestibule of the nose, more comfortable (see Fig. 7.3b). Lower flows, 2–4 L/min, of oxygen are used, which increases the inspired oxygen concentration to 25–40%.

If higher inspired oxygen concentrations are needed in a spontaneously breathing patient, a Hudson mask with a reservoir bag can be used (see Fig. 7.4a). A one-way valve diverts the oxygen flow into the reservoir during expiration. The contents of the reservoir, along with the high flow of oxygen (12–15 L/min) can almost meet the demand of peak inspiration gas flow, resulting in minimal entrainment of air, raising the inspired concentration to approximately 85%. An inspired oxygen concentration of 100% can only be achieved by using either an anaesthetic system with a close-fitting facemask or a self-inflating bag with reservoir and non-rebreathing valve and an oxygen flow of 12–15 L/min.

Fixed-performance devices

These are used when it is important to deliver a precise concentration of oxygen, unaffected by the patient's ventilatory pattern, for example patients with COPD and carbon dioxide retention. These masks work on the principle of high airflow oxygen enrichment (HAFOE). Oxygen is fed into a Venturi that entrains a much greater but constant flow of air. The total flow into the mask should be as high as 45 L/min. The high gas flow has two effects: it meets the patient's peak inspiratory flow, stopping air being drawn in around the mask, and flushes expiratory gas, reducing rebreathing. Masks either deliver a fixed concentration or have interchangeable Venturis to vary the oxygen concentration (Fig. 7.4b).

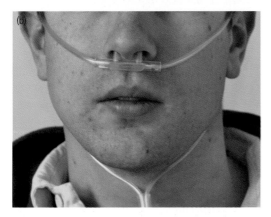

Figure 7.3 (a) Hudson mask. (b) Nasal catheters in position.

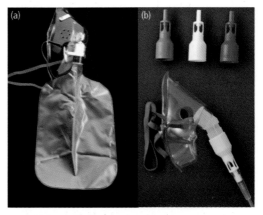

Figure 7.4 (a) Hudson mask with reservoir. (b) High airflow oxygen enrichment (HAFOE; Venturi) mask.

The above systems all deliver dry gas to the patient that may cause crusting or thickening of secretions and difficulty with clearance. For prolonged use, a HAFOE system should be used with a humidifier.

Hypotension

This can be due to a variety of factors, alone or in combination:

- a reduction in circulating volume (preload);
- a reduced cardiac output (reduced myocardial contractility, valvular dysfunction, arrhythmias);
- vasodilatation (afterload).

These should be assessed and treated using a step-wise approach.

Step 1: Assess the circulating volume (preload)

Hypovolaemia is the commonest cause of hypotension after anaesthesia and surgery. Although intraoperative blood loss is usually obvious, continued bleeding, especially in the absence of surgical drains, may not be. Fluid loss may also occur as a result of tissue damage leading to oedema, or from evaporation during prolonged surgery on body cavities, for example the abdomen or thorax (see below). The diagnosis can be confirmed by finding:

- Cold clammy skin, delayed capillary refill (>2 s) in the absence of fear, pain and hypothermia.
- Tachycardia, with a pulse of poor volume.
- Hypotension; initially, systolic blood pressure may be reduced minimally but the diastolic elevated as a result of compensatory vasoconstriction (narrow pulse pressure). The blood pressure must always be interpreted in conjunction with the other assessments.
- Inadequate urine output (<0.5 mL/kg/h), best measured hourly via a catheter and urometer. Consider also the following as causes of reduced urine output:
  ○ a blocked catheter (blood clot or lubricant);
  ○ hypotension;
  ○ hypoxia;
  ○ renal damage intraoperatively (e.g. during aortic aneurysm surgery).

> The commonest cause of oliguria is hypovolaemia; anuria is usually due to a blocked catheter.

The extent to which these changes occur will depend primarily upon the degree of hypovolaemia. A tachycardia may not be seen in the patient taking beta blockers, and a fit, young patient may lose up to 15% of their blood volume without detectable signs.

Treatment

This is covered in detail in Chapter 8.

Step 2: Assess cardiac output

The commonest causes of a reduction in cardiac output are; left ventricular dysfunction due to ischaemic heart disease (or more rarely valvular heart disease) or an arrhythmia.

Left ventricular dysfunction
It is not uncommon to mistake this condition for hypovolaemia based on the presence of poor peripheral circulation, tachycardia and tachypnoeic. However, further examination may reveal:

- distended neck veins, raised JVP;
- basal crepitations on auscultation of the lungs;
- wheeze with a productive cough;
- a triple rhythm on auscultation of the heart.

A chest X-ray may be diagnostic. Echocardiography will demonstrate reduced contractility (hypokinesis) despite adequate ventricular filling suggesting myocardial ischaemia.

Treatment

- Sit the patient upright.
- Give 100% oxygen.
- Monitor the ECG, blood pressure and peripheral oxygen saturation.

Further details are given in Chapter 8.

Arrhythmias
Disturbances of cardiac rhythm are a common cause of hypotension and occur more frequently in the presence of:

- hypoxaemia;
- hypovolaemia;
- hypercarbia;
- hypothermia;
- sepsis;
- pre-existing ischaemic heart disease;
- electrolyte abnormalities;
- acid–base disturbances;
- inotropes, antiarrhythmics, bronchodilators.

Correction of the underlying problem will result in spontaneous resolution of many arrhythmias. Specific intervention is required if there is a significant reduction in cardiac output and hypotension. The management outlined below is based upon the guidelines issued by the Resuscitation Council (UK).

Tachycardias

Cardiac filling occurs during diastole, which is progressively shortened as the heart rate increases. The result is insufficient time for ventricular filling, leading to a reduced cardiac output and eventually a fall in blood pressure. If the contribution from atrial contraction is also lost (for example, in atrial fibrillation) there is further compromise. As coronary artery flow is dependent on diastolic time (and diastolic blood pressure) myocardial ischaemia is more likely particularly in combination with hypotension.

- *Sinus tachycardia (>100 beats/min).* The commonest arrhythmia after anaesthesia and surgery, usually as a result of:
  ○ pain;
  ○ hypovolaemia;
  ○ if there is associated pyrexia, it may be an early indication of sepsis;
  ○ rarely, it may be the first sign of malignant hyperpyrexia.

Treatment consists of oxygen, analgesia and adequate fluid replacement. If the tachycardia persists, a small dose of a beta blocker may be given intravenously whilst monitoring the ECG, providing there are no contraindications.

Treatment of a supraventricular tachycardia (most commonly atrial fibrillation) is covered in Chapter 8.

Bradycardias

Although a slow heart rate reduces myocardial oxygen demand and allows adequate time for ventricular filling, eventually the point is reached where end-diastolic volume is maximal, and further reductions in heart rate reduce cardiac output and hypotension ensues (remember cardiac output = heart rate × stroke volume).

- *Sinus bradycardia (<60 beats/min).* Usually the result of:
  ○ an inadequate dose of an anticholinergic (for instance, glycopyrrolate) given with neostigmine to reverse neuromuscular block;
  ○ excessive suction to clear pharyngeal or tracheal secretions;

○ traction on viscera during surgery;
○ excessive high spread of spinal or epidural anaesthesia;
○ the development of an inferior myocardial infarction;
○ excessive beta-blockade preoperatively or intraoperatively.

Treatment should consist of removing any provoking stimuli and administering oxygen. Further details of treatment are given in Chapter 8.

Step 3: Assess for vasodilatation

This is common during spinal or epidural anaesthesia (see Chapter 5), a typical example being after prostate surgery under spinal anaesthesia. As the legs are taken down from the lithotomy position, vasodilatation in the lower limbs is unmasked, and as the patient is moved to the PACU they become profoundly hypotensive. Hypotension secondary to regional anaesthesia is corrected by giving fluids (crystalloid, colloid), vasopressors (for example, ephedrine), or a combination of both. The combination of hypovolaemia and vasodilatation will cause profound hypotension. Oxygen should always be given.

Sometimes the cause of hypotension is multifactorial as in septic shock where a patient may initially present with peripheral vasodilatation causing hypotension and tachycardia in the absence of blood loss. The patient may be pyrexial and if the cardiac output is measured, it is usually found to be elevated. As sepsis worsens it can lead to reduced cardiac contractility, worsening hypotension, and poor perfusion leading to an acidosis and arrhythmia, often atrial fibrillation. The diagnosis should be suspected in any patient who has had surgery associated with a septic focus, for example free infection in the peritoneal cavity or where there is infection in the genitourinary tract. This usually presents several hours after the patient has left the PACU, often during the night following daytime surgery. The causative micro-organism is often a Gram-negative bacterium. Patients developing septic shock require early diagnosis, invasive monitoring, and circulatory support in a critical care area (see Chapter 8). Antibiotic therapy should be guided by a microbiologist.

> When treating hypotension, correct hypovolaemia before using inotropes.

Hypertension

This is most common in patients with pre-existing hypertension, but may be caused or exacerbated by:

- pain;
- hypoxaemia;
- hypercarbia;
- confusion or delirium;
- hypothermia.

Hypertension with coexisting tachycardia and in the presence of ischaemic heart disease is particularly dangerous as both increase myocardial work and oxygen consumption and may cause an acute myocardial infarction. If the blood pressure remains elevated after correcting the above, a vasodilator or beta blocker may be necessary. Senior help should be sought.

Postoperative nausea and vomiting (PONV)

This occurs in up to 80% of patients following anaesthesia and surgery. It is rarely fatal, but it is unpleasant and leaves patients feeling dissatisfied with the care they have received. Some patients would rather have the pain than the PONV. It may cause delayed discharge from hospital and thereby increase costs. For these reasons it is to be taken seriously and measures should be employed to avoid it.

Patients identified as being at risk of PONV should be given an anti-emetic before emergence from anaesthesia because it is often easier to prevent vomiting than to stop it once it has started. Failure of treatment may be addressed in the PACU by giving a second or third drug from the different classes (see Chapter 3).

Most PACUs have a PONV pathway to ensure optimal management of patients at risk (Fig. 7.5).

Postoperative intravenous fluid therapy

A 70 kg man is composed of approximately 45 L of water, of which 30 L are in the intracellular space and 15 L in the extracellular space. The latter is divided into the interstitial space (10 L) and the intravascular space (5 L). Daily water intake is of approximately 2500 mL comprising; 1500 mL orally, 750 mL in food and 250 mL generated by the oxidation of carbohydrates. A similar volume is lost each day; 1500 mL as urine, 100 mL in faeces and 900 mL as insensible losses (300 mL via the lungs, 600 mL via the skin). To maintain electrolyte balance the following intake is required; sodium 1–1.5 mmol/kg, potassium 1 mmol/kg and 0.1–0.2 mmol/kg each of calcium, magnesium and phosphate. Inadequate water intake is sensed by osmo- and volume receptors that stimulate the release of antidiuretic hormone (ADH) and the sensation of thirst.

Minor surgery

All patients having an anaesthetic (and surgery) undergo a period of fasting pre- and intraoperatively, resulting in a water deficit. The loss comes from the total body water (intra and extracellular fluid), which therefore has little effect on the intravascular volume. This is well tolerated when surgery is relatively minor and there is no significant blood loss. Providing that such patients resume oral intake 1–2 hours postoperatively, they do not routinely need IV fluid in the perioperative period. The only exceptions to this are children and the elderly who are very intolerant of even relatively minor degrees of dehydration and those patients with a high risk of PONV, where giving fluids may reduce the risk.

If surgery is prolonged, or a patient has failed to drink within 4–6 hours of recovering from anaesthesia, usually as a result of nausea and vomiting, IV fluid will be required. Providing that the volume of vomit is not excessive, only maintenance fluids are required. These are calculated at 1.5 mL/kg/h, but must take into account the accrued deficit.

For example, a 70 kg patient fasted from 08:00 to 14:00, who is still unable to take fluids by mouth at 18:00 will require:

- 1.5 mL/kg/h to make up the deficit from 08:00 to 18:00

$$= 1.5 \times 70 \text{ (kg)} \times 10 \text{ (h)} = 1000 \text{ mL};$$

- 1.5 mL/kg/h from 18:00 to 08:00 the following morning

$$= 1.5 \times 70 \text{ (kg)} \times 14 \text{ (h)} = 1400 \text{ mL}.$$

The total IV fluid requirement = 2400 mL in the next 14 h if they are not able to resume

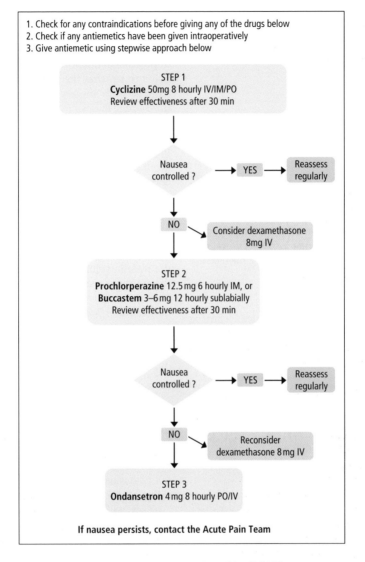

1. Check for any contraindications before giving any of the drugs below
2. Check if any antiemetics have been given intraoperatively
3. Give antiemetic using stepwise approach below

STEP 1
Cyclizine 50mg 8 hourly IV/IM/PO
Review effectiveness after 30 min

Nausea controlled ? → YES → Reassess regularly

NO → Consider dexamethasone 8mg IV

STEP 2
Prochlorperazine 12.5mg 6 hourly IM, or
Buccastem 3–6mg 12 hourly sublabially
Review effectiveness after 30 min

Nausea controlled ? → YES → Reassess regularly

NO → Reconsider dexamethasone 8mg IV

STEP 3
Ondansetron 4mg 8 hourly PO/IV

If nausea persists, contact the Acute Pain Team

Figure 7.5 Treatment pathway for postoperative nausea and vomiting (PONV).

oral intake. An appropriate rate for the IV fluid would be:

- 1000 mL over the first 4 hours;
- 1000 mL over the following 6 hours;
- 500 mL over the last 4 hours.

This should contain the daily requirement of Na 1–1.5 mmol/kg and could be given either as:

- 2 × 1000 mL 5% glucose plus 500 mL 0.9% (normal) saline; or

- 2 × 1000 mL 4% glucose/0.18% saline, plus 500 mL 4% glucose/0.18% saline.

In practice most patients would probably be prescribed fluid at the rate of 1000 mL per 8 hours either as 0.9% saline or Hartmann's solution. Clearly this contains a greater amount of sodium than required but this is easily excreted by the kidneys. Whatever regime is prescribed, patients should be reviewed at 22:00 and 08:00 the following morning to ensure that they are adequately hydrated (see below).

Major surgery

Postoperative fluid balance following major surgery is more complex. Assuming that appropriate volumes of water, electrolytes and blood have been given during the operation, the postoperative fluid and electrolyte requirements will depend upon:

- the volume needed for maintenance, which will be increased if the patient is pyrexial;
- replacement of continuing losses from the gastrointestinal tract, for example via a nasogastric tube, fistulae, diarrhoea;
- losses into drains;
- any continued bleeding;
- rewarming of cold peripheries causing vasodilatation;
- the presence of an epidural for analgesia;
- the extent of tissue trauma or 'third space losses'.

No single regime can cover all eventualities. The most important factor is clinical assessment and reassessment, along with appropriate monitoring. Further advice is available from GIFTASUP (see useful information section).

Third space losses

The first and second spaces are the constituents of the ECF, namely the interstitial fluid space and the plasma. These are normal physiological compartments and fluid shifts occur readily between them. A 'third space' related to and formed from the ECF also exists and in non-pathological circumstances is usually referred to as the transcellular water, examples being CSF, urine, fluid within the gut, and fluids in the ducts of glands and serous cavities. Accumulation of third-space fluid may also be pathological, examples being the swelling of tissues after surgical trauma or burns, ascites, pleural effusions and fluid within the bowel lumen in a patient who has an ileus. In health, fluid intake replenishes the ECF, but in pathological conditions, the interstitial and plasma fluid volumes become depleted in proportion to the volume of the third-space losses. This has a proportionately greater effect on the plasma

volume than if the losses were distributed from the total body water, for example in dehydration. The biggest problem for the clinician is that it is impossible to quantify such losses accurately, suffice it to say that the greater the degree of tissue damage from surgery or trauma, the greater the third-space losses.

The patient who has undergone major surgery will require close monitoring to ensure that sufficient volumes of the correct fluid are given to replace what has been lost. These losses can be divided into two main groups; those that equate to ECF (blood, losses from the GI tract, third space losses) and those that are mainly water (insensible losses). As seen above, the former will have a greater immediate effect as a significant part of the loss is from the plasma volume, and consequently will affect the perfusion and oxygenation of vital organs. This must be rectified rapidly. As already mentioned water losses, unless excessive, have less of an effect on circulating volume and can be replaced more gradually.

In the first 24 hours postoperatively, no single regime can be provided, but the following must be taken into account when calculating and prescribing fluid therapy for each individual patient:

- Maintenance fluids
  - 1.5 mL/kg/h water, increased by 10% for each °C if the patient is pyrexial;
  - sodium, 1–1.5 mmol/kg;
  - potassium 1.0 mmol/kg;
- Replacement of measured gastrointestinal losses with an equal volume of Hartmann's solution.
- Replacement of ongoing blood loss. Aim for a haemoglobin concentration of 9.0 g/dl.
  - <500 mL with either Hartmann's solution or 0.9% saline (up to three times the volume of blood lost as crystalloids are distributed throughout the ECF), or colloid, to the same volume as the blood loss;
  - >1000 mL may require transfusion with stored blood.
- Replacement of ongoing losses into the third space.
- Fluid required as a result of epidural induced vasodilatation.

Patients that have undergone major body cavity surgery may require large volumes of fluid postoperatively. In order to ensure that their demands are met they must be regularly assessed, clinically, biochemically, and by the use of invasive monitoring, where appropriate.

Clinical assessment

- Thirst, dry mucous membranes; early reliable signs of dehydration.
- Cool peripheries, reduced skin turgor, tachycardia, oliguria, drowsiness; implies a significant fluid deficit.
- Hypotension, increased respiratory rate, coma; life threatening.
- Urine output, less than 0.5 mL/kg/hr suggests significant hypovolaemia.

A review of the patient's observation charts looking at trends is often more useful than a 'snapshot' of their condition. Deterioration suggests that treatment is inadequate or that there are new or ongoing unidentified problems.

Biochemistry

- Raised haematocrit, urea, creatinine; support the diagnosis of dehydration.
- Metabolic acidosis; suggests hypovolaemia and hypoperfusion.

Monitoring

Central venous pressure is normally 2–5 mmHg (3–8 cmH$_2$O); a low or negative CVP indicates fluid depletion. Trends are more useful, particularly the response to a fluid challenge; 250 mL fluid are given rapidly and the change in CVP noted. In a hypovolaemic patient there will be a brief increase followed by a fall to the previous value. When the circulating volume is adequate there will be a small sustained rise. Overtransfusion will be seen as a high, sustained CVP. Increasingly, stroke volume and cardiac output are optimized using non-invasive methods of monitoring (see Chapter 2).

On the second and subsequent days, the same basic principles are used. In addition:

- the fluid balance of the previous 24 h must be checked;
- ensure that all sources of fluid loss are recorded;
- the patient's serum electrolytes must be checked to ensure adequate replacement and the fluid regime should be adjusted accordingly;

- the urine output for the previous 6 and 24 hours should be noted; if decreasing, consider other causes of fluid loss, such increasing pyrexia or development of an ileus;
- magnesium and phosphate levels must be checked and replacements given if plasma concentration are low;
- consider starting enteral nutrition, either orally or via a nasogastric tube.

The stress response

Following major surgery and trauma, matters are complicated further. Various neuroendocrine responses result in an increased secretion of a variety of hormones, which have an effect on fluid balance. Antidiuretic hormone (ADH) secretion is maximal during surgery and may remain elevated for several days. The effect of this is to increase water absorption by the kidneys and reduce urine output. Aldosterone secretion is raised and together with activation of the renin–angiotensin system results in sodium and fluid retention and increased urinary excretion of potassium. Consequently, in some patients, urine output may be as low as 0.5 mL/kg per hour during the first two postoperative days without signifying organ hypoperfusion. Furthermore they will not have the clinical signs associated with dehydration (see Chapter 8). Additional fluid, in an attempt to restore urine output is unnecessary and simply leads to greater sodium and water retention, worsening tissue oedema without producing an increase in urine output. This is particularly true after pulmonary and oesophageal surgery, where it has been shown that maintaining normal fluid input and accepting a lower urine output results in fewer postoperative complications, as a result of less tissue oedema and fewer anastamotic breakdowns. It is important to remember that all clinical parameters need to be considered when trying to judge intravascular volume and tissue perfusion. However, in some cases where there are on-going 'third space' losses, for example after major trauma, patients will exhibit clinical symptoms and signs of fluid depletion and increased IV fluids will be required to maintain an adequate intravascular volume.

After 3–5 days, hormone levels return to normal and this is followed by an increase in the volume of urine passed, which may be augmented as fluid sequestered to the pathological third space is reclaimed.

Postoperative analgesia

After injury, acute pain limits activity until healing has taken place. Modern surgical treatment restores function more rapidly, a process facilitated by the elimination of postoperative pain. A good example is the internal fixation of fractures, followed by potent analgesia allowing early mobilization. Ineffective treatment of postoperative pain not only delays this process, but also has other important consequences:

- physical immobility:
  - reduced cough, sputum retention and pneumonia;
  - muscle wasting, skin breakdown and cardiovascular deconditioning;
  - thromboembolic disease – deep venous thrombosis and pulmonary embolus;
  - delayed bone and soft tissue healing;
- psychological reaction:
  - reluctance to undergo further, necessary surgical procedures;
- economic costs:
  - prolonged hospital stay, increased medical complications;
  - increased time away from normal occupations;
- development of chronic pain syndromes.

Sometimes pain is a useful aid to diagnosis and must be recognized and acted upon, for example:

- pain due to a compartment syndrome;
- pain caused by, dressings becoming too tight;
- pain of infection from cellulitis, peritonitis or pneumonia;
- referred visceral pain in myocardial infarction (arm or neck) or pancreatitis (to the back).

> Any patient who complains of pain that unexpectedly increases in severity, changes in nature or site, or is of new onset should be examined to identify the cause rather than simply be prescribed analgesia.

Factors affecting the experience of pain

Pain and the patient's response to it are very variable and should be understood against the background of the individual's previous personal experiences and expectations rather than compared with the norm:

- Anxiety heightens the experience of pain. The preoperative visit by the anaesthetist plays a significant role in allaying anxiety by explaining what to expect postoperatively, what types of analgesia are available and also by exploring patients concerns with them.
- Patients who have a pre-existing chronic pain problem are vulnerable to suffering with additional acute pain. Their nervous systems can be considered to be sensitized to pain and will react more strongly to noxious stimuli. Bad previous pain experiences in hospital or anticipation of severe pain for another reason suggest that extra effort will be required to control the pain.
- Older patients tend to require lower doses of analgesics as a result of changes in drug distribution, metabolism, excretion, and coexisting disease. Prescribing should take these factors into account rather than using them as an excuse for inadequate analgesia. There is no difference between the intensity of pain suffered by the different sexes having the same operation.
- Upper abdominal and thoracic surgery cause the most severe pain of the longest duration, control of which is important because of the detrimental effects on ventilation. Pain following surgery on the body wall or periphery of limbs is less severe and for a shorter duration.

Management of postoperative pain

This can be divided into a number of steps:

- assessment of pain;
- analgesic drugs used;
- techniques of administration;
- difficult pain problems.

Assessment of acute pain

Regular measurement of pain means that it is less likely to be ignored and the efficacy of interventions can be assessed. There are a variety of methods of assessing pain; Table 7.3 shows a simple, practical system that is understood by patients and easily applied by staff. The numeric score is to facilitate recording and allows trends to be

Table 7.3 A simple practical scoring system for acute pain

Pain score	Staff view	Patient's view	Action
0	None	Insignificant or no pain	Consider reducing dose or changing to weaker analgesic, e.g. morphine to NSAID plus paracetamol
1	Mild	In pain, but expected and tolerable; no reason to seek (additional) treatment	Continue current therapy, review regularly
2	Moderate	Unpleasant situation; treatment desirable but not necessarily at the expense of severe treatment side effects	Continue current therapy, consider additional regular simple analgesia, e.g. paracetamol and/or NSAID
3	Severe	Intolerable situation – will consider even unpleasant treatments to reduce pain	Increase dose of opioid, or start opioid; consider alternative technique, e.g. epidural

identified. Pain must be assessed with appropriate activity for the stage of recovery; for example, five days after a hip joint replacement, a patient would not be expected to have pain while lying in bed, but adequate analgesia should allow mobilization with only mild to insignificant pain.

Analgesic drugs used postoperatively

The most commonly used drugs are opioids, NSAIDs and local anaesthetics. Their sites of action are shown in Fig. 7.6.

Opioids
The pharmacology of opioid drugs and their side-effects are covered in Chapter 3. In the UK, morphine is widely used to control severe postoperative pain on surgical units and can be given by several routes (Table 7.4). One of the principal metabolites, morphine-6-glucuronide (M6G), has potent opioid effects and may accumulate and cause toxicity in patients with renal failure, particularly the elderly. Fentanyl and oxycodone have less active metabolites than morphine, and have faster onset of action, so may be more suitable for these patients.

For most painful clinical conditions there will be a blood level of opioid that provides useful analgesia, that is, a reduction in pain level. The dose required to achieve this may vary enormously between patients as a result of differences in the following:

- Pharmacodynamics: the effect of the drug on the body (via the receptors).
- Pharmacokinetics: how the body distributes, metabolizes and eliminates the drug.

- The nature of the stimulus.
- The psychological reaction to the situation.

The biggest step forward in the treatment of acute pain with opioids has been the recognition that individual requirements are very variable and the dose needs to be titrated for each patient:

- there is no minimum or maximum dose;
- even with best practice some pain will remain;
- minimum levels of monitoring and intervention are necessary for safe and effective use;
- use a multimodal approach to minimize the dose of opioids and thereby side effects;
- additional methods of analgesia should be considered if opioid requirements are high.

Overdose
Profound respiratory depression and coma due to opioids must be treated using the ABC principles described in Chapter 8. Having created a patent airway and supported ventilation using a bag-valve-mask with supplementary oxygen, the effects of the opioid can be pharmacologically reversed (antagonized). Naloxone (0.4 mg) is diluted to 5 mL with 0.9% saline and given in incremental doses of 1 mL IV (adult dosing). Analgesia will also be reversed, and careful thought must be given to continuing analgesia. In this situation, HDU care is usually advisable.

Long-term complications of opioids
Adequate treatment of acute pain with opioids is not associated with dependency.

Non-steroidal anti-inflammatory drugs (NSAIDs)
The pharmacology of these drugs is covered in Chapter 3.

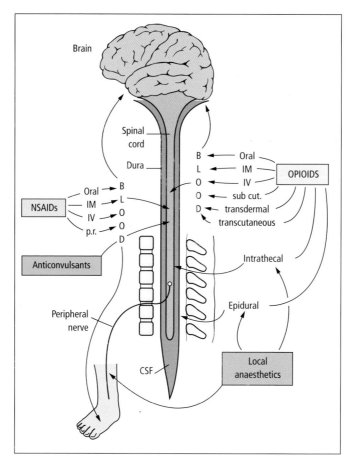

Figure 7.6 Sites of actions of analgesic drugs.

Analgesic techniques used postoperatively

Patient-controlled analgesia (PCA)

- A microprocessor-controlled syringe pump capable of being programmed is used to deliver a predetermined dose of a drug intravenously.
- Activation is by the patient depressing a switch that is designed to prevent accidental triggering (hence 'patient-controlled').

To prevent the administration of an overdose:

- The maximum dose in any period and any background infusion is predetermined.
- After successful administration of a dose, a subsequent dose cannot be given for a preset period, the 'lockout period'.
- Typical settings for an adult using morphine delivered by a PCA device might be:
  - ○ bolus dose: 1 mg;
  - ○ lockout interval: 5 min.
- PCA devices record attempts made by the patient to access analgesia, allowing the dose to be adjusted to meet their requirements.

Effective PCA requires:

- The patient to be briefed by the anaesthetist and/or nursing staff preoperatively and, if possible, be shown the device to be used.
- A loading dose of analgesic, usually intravenously before starting. Failure to do this will result in the patient being unable to get sufficient analgesia from the PCA device and the system will fail.
- A dedicated IV cannula or non-return valve on an IV infusion to prevent accumulation of the drug and failure of analgesia.

Table 7.4 Morphine preparations

Oral	Immediate release (IR) tablets or liquid: • Absorption and effect within minutes • Usual adult dose 20 mg hourly prn • Less in elderly, more if opioid tolerant • Providing the gut is working, useful even after major surgery • Usually used for acute pain where the opioid requirement is unknown or changing rapidly Modified release (MR) tablets, capsules or granules: • Dose released over either 12 or 24 hours • Avoids frequent dosing with immediate release preparations • Useful when opioid requirement is prolonged and also for gradually weaning down the dose at the end of treatment The two formulations are usually used together to provide a steady background level of analgesa (MR) with additional breakthrough doses (IR) as required *It is important that everybody understands the difference between MR and IR forms of morphine*
Intravenous	Morphine 10 or 20 mg diluted to 1 mg/mL with 0.9% sodium chloride can be given: • In increments initially of 1–3 mg at 3 min intervals; effective dose may range from 1 to 50 mg or more (the latter in opioid-tolerant patients) • Via patient controlled analgesia device (see text) • As a continuous infusion. Useful where patient cooperation is limited, e.g. in elderly patients or ITU. Problems occur in predicting the correct infusion rate, given the variability of dose requirement between patients. Very close supervision is required to avoid underinfusion (pain) or overinfusion (toxicity). This method can be used to replace high doses of oral opioids during the perioperative period *The intravenous dose of morphine is about one-third of the oral dose*
Intramuscular	A predetermined dose (e.g. morphine 10 mg) at fixed minimum intervals, e.g. hourly • Delayed and variable rate of effect • Precise titration is difficult with repeated cycles of pain and relief • Does not require complex equipment or a cooperative patient • Although widely available, gradually being replaced by the above

• Observation and recording of the patient's pain score, sedation score, and respiratory rate is essential to ensure success. Any patient with a respiratory rate less than 8 breaths/min and a sedation score of 2 or 3 requires immediate intervention:
  ○ stop the PCA;
  ○ give oxygen via a mask;
  ○ call for assistance;
  ○ consider giving naloxone (see above);
  ○ if the patient is apnoeic, commence ventilation using a self-inflating bag-valve-mask device.

Advantages of PCA

• Greater flexibility; analgesia matched to the patient's perception of the pain.
• Reduced workload for the nursing staff.
• Elimination of painful IM injections.
• Drug given IV with greater certainty of adequate plasma levels.

Disadvantages

• Equipment is expensive to purchase and maintain.
• It requires patient comprehension of the system.
• Patient must be physically able to trigger the device.
• The elderly are often reluctant to use a PCA device.
• The potential for overdose if the device is incorrectly programmed.

As pain subsides the PCA can be discontinued, and oral analgesics can be used. The first dose should be given 1 hour prior to discontinuing PCA, to ensure continuity of analgesia.

Regional analgesic techniques (Fig. 7.7)

• *Peripheral nerve blocks.* Used mainly for pain relief after upper or lower limb surgery. A single

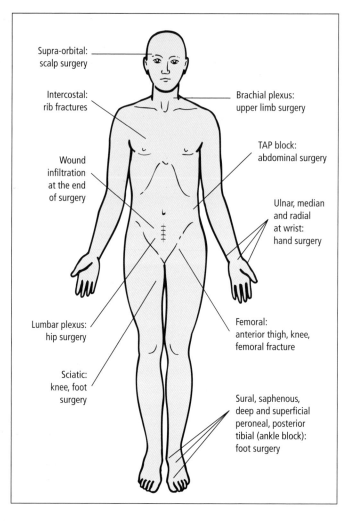

Supra-orbital:
scalp surgery

Intercostal:
rib fractures

Wound
infiltration
at the end
of surgery

Brachial plexus:
upper limb surgery

TAP block:
abdominal surgery

Ulnar, median
and radial
at wrist:
hand surgery

Lumbar plexus:
hip surgery

Sciatic:
knee, foot
surgery

Femoral:
anterior thigh, knee,
femoral fracture

Sural, saphenous,
deep and superficial
peroneal, posterior
tibial (ankle block):
foot surgery

Figure 7.7 Some commonly used nerve blocks.

injection of local anaesthetic, usually bupivacaine, results in 6–12 hours of pain relief. An infusion of local anaesthetic via a catheter inserted close to the nerve may enable the block to be continued for several days. An alternative and effective form of analgesia must be prescribed for when the local anaesthetic is discontinued to prevent the patient being in severe pain.

- *Transverus abdominis plane (TAP) block (see also Chapter 5).* Infusion of local anaesthetic via a catheter placed in the plane between the transversus abdominis and internal oblique muscles to anaesthetise the nerves supplying the skin and muscles of the anterior abdominal wall (and parietal peritoneum).

- *Epidural analgesia (see also Chapter 5).* Infusions of a local anaesthetic into the epidural space, either alone or in combination with opioids, act on the transiting nerve roots and the dorsal horn of the spinal cord, respectively, to provide dramatic relief of postoperative pain. It is essential that patients who are offered an epidural receive an explanation by the anaesthetist at the preoperative visit of what to expect postoperatively, in particular altered sensation, weakness of the lower limbs, and the potential need for a urinary catheter. The epidural is often sited preoperatively and used intraoperatively as part of the anaesthetic technique. For upper abdominal surgery an epidural in the mid-thoracic region (T6/7) is used, while a hip operation would need a lumbar epidural (L1/2).

Different combinations of local anaesthetic and opioid infusion have been used successfully. Ideally, the concentration of local anaesthetic should selectively block sensory nerves, with relative sparing of motor nerves. The choice and dose of opioid should be such that the drug passes through the dura into the CSF in sufficient quantities to block the opioid receptors in the spinal cord but not spread cranially to cause respiratory depression, for example bupivacaine 0.125% plus fentanyl 2–4 µg/mL. Epidural infusions can be used to maintain analgesia for several days. Opioid side-effects are less common and less severe than when given systemically as the dose is much less.

There are a number of important points to bear in mind when using epidural analgesia:

- The infusion rate and the site of the catheter determine the spread of the solution. In the thoracic epidural space a starting infusion rate might be 4 mL/h; in the lumbar space commence at 8 mL/h.
- The efficacy of the infusion must be monitored in a similar manner as for PCA.
- If analgesia is inadequate, a 'top-up' of 3–4 mL of solution may be necessary.
- Observations of the patient's vital signs should then be made on a regular basis according to local protocol.
- In patients over the age of 60 years, the concentration of opioid is often halved.

Management of complications during postoperative epidural analgesia

Epidurals are commonly used for analgesia during labour and in the early postoperative period following abdominal or thoracic surgery. The aim is to 'block' all of the nerve roots which carry sensory nerves from the area of tissue injury. They are usually run as a continuous infusion of low-dose local anaesthetic and an opioid (for example, 0.1% levo-bupicacaine and 2 µg/ml fentanyl) controlled by a dedicated infusion pump, but at times may require a bolus dose to improve the quality of analgesia. The complications arising as a result of the use of local anaesthetics are the same as when they are used intraoperatively, and are covered in Chapter 5. All patients having epidural analgesia require regular monitoring and documentation of:

- heart rate and blood pressure;
- respiratory rate and peripheral oxygen saturations;
- urine output;
- pain scores at rest and on movement;
- lower limb motor function;
- conscious level, usually assessed using the Glasgow Coma Scale (GCS) score.

As a general rule, any complications related to an epidural should be discussed with an anaesthetist, or the hospital's acute pain team. There are a number of complications that may present whilst a patient is receiving epidural analgesia or after it has been stopped, including:

- *Hypotension*. Due to block of the sympathetic nerves:
  - block of T2–L2 results in vasodilatation, a drop in systemic vascular resistance, and hypotension;
  - block of the thoracic nerve roots above T5 also reduces heart rate and contractility;
  - patients with additional fluid losses, for example haemorrhage, are particularly vulnerable to severe hypotension;
  - the legs can be raised to counteract the vasodilatation, the equivalent to a 500 mL fluid challenge;
  - a fluid bolus, for example 500 mL Hartmann's should be given immediately; a vasopressor can also be given, for example ephedrine 3–6 mg IV;
  - a bradycardia with 'adverse features' should be treated with atropine 500 µg IV;
  - the extent of the block should be checked, the epidural infusion may need to be stopped or the rate reduced, and an anaesthetist called urgently to plan further management;
  - the patient may need admission to a critical care area for close monitoring as the effect of the epidural anaesthetic already given may last for several hours.
- *Respiratory depression*. Due to either systemic absorption of the opioid or secondary to block of the thoracic nerve roots:

○ highly lipid soluble opioids (diamorphine, fentanyl) are rapidly taken up by the spinal cord, limiting their spread and systemic absorption, and respiratory depression tends to occur early; less soluble opioids (morphine) are taken up slowly, and respiratory depression tends to occur later;

○ motor block above T4 will paralyse the intercostal muscles, impairing ventilation;

○ evaluation of the block height and risk factors for opioid sensitivity will help determine which is most likely;

○ in either case, stop the epidural infusion, at least temporarily;

○ if opioid narcosis is suspected, give 100–200 µg of naloxone IV;

○ support ventilation if necessary;

○ seek expert help.

- *Urinary retention.* Due to both the loss of the sensation of a full bladder and the direct effect of opioids on the sphincter muscles:
  ○ more common in males, particularly if there are already symptoms of prostatism;
  ○ urinary retention usually results in complete anuria, and the bladder may be palpable in the supra-pubic area of the abdomen;
  ○ oliguria is more likely to be due to hypotension or hypovolaemia, other intra-abdominal pathology, and needs appropriate management depending on the cause;
  ○ it may be prevented by routine monitoring of urine output in all postoperative patients;
  ○ it may require short-term catheterization.

- *Motor block (leg weakness).* This is most common when concentrated local anaesthetic solutions (0.25% or 0.5% levo-bupivacaine) are used; it is less frequent with low concentrations (0.1% levo-bupivacaine):
  ○ it may lead to pressure ulcers on the patient's heels or sacrum due to lack of movement, or falls whilst mobilizing;
  ○ the infusion should be stopped and anaesthetic/pain team informed;
  ○ it may be prevented by regular observation of effects of epidural and correct adjustment of infusion rate.

Worsening or severe leg weakness is not a normal feature of epidural analgesia and needs investigating urgently. Possible causes include:

- Intrathecal migration of the epidural catheter – the local anaesthetic is then delivered intrathecally causing an extensive spinal.

- Epidural haematoma – the risk is greater in patients on anticoagulants, antiplatelet drugs, those with a coagulopathy or thrombocytopenia.

- Epidural abscess – an infection introduced via the catheter, which is more common with prolonged use of an epidural:
  ○ haematomas and abscesses can produce symptoms after the catheter has been removed;
  ○ patients complain typically of increasing back pain;
  ○ this may be delayed for several weeks so that the connection to the surgery and epidural may be missed (up to several weeks later in the case of abscess!).
  ○ If an epidural haematoma or abscess is suspected the investigation of choice is urgent MR scanning.

- Damage to nerves or the spinal cord during insertion of the needle and systemic toxicity of the local *anaesthetic*. These are both unusual complications.

- *Inadequate analgesia.* This is usually a consequence of inadequate spread of the local anaesthetic solution to all nerve roots:
  ○ a bolus dose of local anaesthetic may be required and the rate of infusion may need to be increased – this should be done by an anaesthetist familiar with epidural analgesia;
  ○ there may be pain for sites not covered by the epidural, for example pain referred to the shoulder due to diaphragmatic irritation:
    - it may require alterative systemic analgesia;
    - systemic opioids should not be given if the epidural solution contains an opioid.

- *Pruritus.* This can be severe and frequently localized to the nose; it may respond to antihistamines, atropine or naloxone.

- *Headache.* This occurs in 0.5–1% of epidurals, due to puncture of the dura by the needle (or catheter) and subsequent CSF leak. This is often referred to as a 'post dural puncture headache' (PDPH).
  ○ it may or may not be recognized at the time of performing the epidural;
  ○ it typically develops 24–48 hours after epidural insertion and is worse on sitting or standing and better on lying down;
  ○ an anaesthetist should be informed, who can assess the patient and discuss appropriate management, possibly an epidural 'blood patch';

○ many headaches respond well to simple measures such as paracetamol, NSAIDs and good fluid intake encouraged.

> *Any* patient with an epidural, who develops increasing motor blockade in the absence of excessive anaesthetic doses, needs to be reviewed by a senior anaesthetist.

Intrathecal (spinal) analgesia

Spinal anaesthesia is of insufficient duration to provide postoperative pain relief. However, if a small dose of opioid, for example diamorphine 250–500 µg, is injected along with the local anaesthetic, this may provide 12–24 hours of analgesia. Complications are the same as those due to opioids given epidurally and are managed in the same way.

Other techniques

Entonox is a mixture of nitrous oxide (50%) and oxygen (50%). It is a weak analgesic with sedative properties and is useful for short-term analgesia for painful procedures, such as change of dressings. It should be avoided in patients with a pneumothorax because the nitrous oxide may diffuse into the gas-filled space, increasing the volume.

Combining analgesic techniques

Examples of good practice are:

- bupivacaine and fentanyl in an epidural infusion;
- intravenous PCA morphine and intravenous paracoxib in the early postoperative period when patients are nil by mouth;
- oral morphine immediate release (IR) tablets and paracetamol prescribed to be given as a spinal wears off.

Difficult pain problems

Patients who show evidence of regular opioid use preoperatively, such as drug addicts, cancer and chronic pain patients and those patients with a previous bad pain experience, may pose a particular problem postoperatively. They are best managed if they are identified at the preoperative assessment and a team approach is used that will include:

- liaison with the acute pain team to inform them of the patient's admission;
- discussion with the anaesthetist, and surgical and nursing staff to plan perioperative care, to:

○ ensure any current opioid medication is continued on admission to prevent withdrawal;
○ understand that much larger doses of opioids than normal may be required;
○ explain that toxicity from high doses of opioid is very unlikely;
○ reassure that addiction is not a concern;
- discussion with the patient to explain:
○ types and effectiveness of analgesic regimes available postoperatively;
○ that analgesia may not be 100% effective;
○ that long-term continuation may be necessary;
○ potential side effects, especially if regional analgesia planned;
- plan regular reviews during postoperative period;
- coordination of care.

FURTHER USEFUL INFORMATION

Bay I, Nunn JF, Prys Roberts C. Factors affecting arterial PO_2 during recovery from general anaesthesia. *British Journal of Anaesthesia* 1968; **40**: 398–407.

Gan TJ, Meyer T, Apfel CC *et al*. Consensus guidelines for managing postoperative nausea and vomiting. *Anesthesia and Analgesia* 2003; **97**: 62–71.

Good Practice in the Management of Epidural Analgesia in the Hospital Setting. The Royal College of Anaesthetists. 2004, http://www.rcoa.ac.uk/docs/EpiduralAnalgesia2010.pdf

O'Driscoll BR, Howard LS, Davison AG; British Thoracic Society. The British Thoracic Society guideline for emergency oxygen use in adult patients. *Thorax* 2008; **63** (supplement VI): vi1–vi68.

Powell-Tuck J, Gosling P, Lobo DN *et al*. *British consensus guidelines on intravenous fluid therapy for adult surgical patients (GIFTASUP)*. London: NHS Library of Health, www.renal.org/pages/media/download_gallery/GIFTASUP%20FINAL_05_01_09.pdf.

Thomson AJ, Webb DJ, Maxwell SRJ, Grant IS. Oxygen therapy in acute medical care. *British Medical Journal* 2002; **324**: 1406–7.

West JB. *Respiratory physiology: the essentials*, 9th edn. Baltimore: Williams & Wilkins, 2011.

www.aagbi.org/publications/guidelines/docs/postanaes02.pdf
[Immediate postanaesthetic recovery. The Association of Anaesthetists of Great Britain & Ireland. September 2002.]

www.asahq.org/publicationsAndServices/practiceparam.htm

[Numerous practice guidelines by the American Society of Anesthesiologists on a variety of topics, one of which is post-anaesthetic care.]

www.medicine.ox.ac.uk/bandolier/booth/pain-pag/index2.html

[The Oxford Pain site. Brilliant for the latest evidence-based information on all aspects of acute pain.]

http://oac.med.jhmi.edu/res_phys/

[The Johns Hopkins School of Medicine interactive respiratory physiology website.]

www.rcoa.ac.uk/docs/ARB-section3.pdf

[Audit topics and useful information about postoperative care from The Royal College of Anaesthetists.]

www.resus.org.uk/pages/periarst.pdf

[Current Resuscitation Council UK guidelines on peri-arrest arrhythmias.]

All websites last accessed February 2012.

? SELF-ASSESSMENT

Short-answer questions

7.1 List the three main causes of hypoxaemia immediately postoperatively and give examples of a cause of each. What devices could be used to treat this problem and what concentration of oxygen will each deliver?

7.2 What are the three main causes of hypotension in the immediate postoperative period? What would be your immediate management?

7.3 Calculate the fluid requirement for the next 24 hours in a 60-year-old man at 09:00, who had a laparotomy the previous afternoon. He weighs 80 kg and is apyrexial. His BP is 95/65 mmHg, pulse rate 110/min and he is complaining of feeling thirsty. In the last 12 hours he has passed 340 ml urine and lost 400 ml via a nasogastric tube. His serum sodium is 137 mmol/l, potassium 3.2 mmol/l and Hb 7.2 g/dl.

7.4 Describe how a patient controlled analgesia (PCA) device works. What are the advantages and disadvantages of such a device?

7.5 What are the common complications resulting from the use of an epidural for postoperative analgesia and how are they treated?

True/false questions

7.1 Ventilation/perfusion mismatch:
  a is increased postoperatively due to areas of atelectasis;
  b resulting in V/Q > 1 is the equivalent of dead space;
  c Resulting in V/Q = 0 is the equivalent of a shunt;
  d Is common in the obese and the elderly postoperatively.

7.2 Under normal circumstances:
  a two-thirds of the total body water is intra-cellular;
  b the daily requirement of water is 3 mL/kg/h;
  c 2000 mL of normal (0.9%) saline provides the daily requirement of sodium and chloride;
  d the daily requirement of potassium is approximately 1 mmol/kg.

7.3 The following are features of the stress response following major surgery:
  a decreased anti-diuretic hormone (ADH) production;
  b increased circulating aldosterone levels;
  c increased urine production;
  d inevitable AKI.

7.4 When considering postoperative analgesia:
  a patient requirements are very variable;
  b good pain control can reduce morbidity and mortality;
  c multi-modal regimes are best avoided as interactions and side effects are more common;
  d it is not possible for a patient to overdose using a PCA device.

7.5 Complications of epidural analgesia include:
  a poor urine output;
  b pruritis;
  c headache;
  d leg weakness.

The acutely ill adult patient on the ward

> **Tips for anaesthesia attachments**
>
> During your time in anaesthesia, try to spend time on the ITU and with the team that responds to emergencies on the ward and participate in the:
>
> - systematic assessment and treatment of a critically ill patient;
> - initial management of some common life-threatening emergencies:
>   - airway obstruction;
>   - acute shortness of breath;
>   - shock;
>   - arrhythmia or cardiac arrest;
>   - acute kidney injury;
>   - impaired consciousness.

Section 1: Recognition and assessment

The focus of this chapter is on how to recognize and initially manage acute problems commonly encountered on general hospital wards and how to refer such patients effectively to senior colleagues if there is not a prompt improvement in the patient's condition in response to initial management. All too often, misinterpretation of the clinical picture may lead either to a lack of action or to treatment being commenced that is inappropriate. A classic anecdotal example is the elderly post-operative patient who is breathless, hypotensive, oliguric and has crackles on auscultation of the chest. Acute heart failure is diagnosed and a large dose of an intravenous diuretic is given. The correct diagnosis may in fact be pneumonia, sepsis and pre-renal failure secondary to hypovolaemia and hypotension. Although the intravenous diuretic may initially increase urine output, ultimately it will exacerbate the dehydration and pre-renal failure, and may even precipitate acute cardiovascular collapse.

The immediate aim is to identify dysfunction in one or more organ systems and initiate appropriate treatment to prevent further deterioration before frank organ system failure supervenes. Once this has been achieved, appropriate investigations will help to make a clinical diagnosis of the cause of the patient's illness. Even if this is not possible, early referral for higher level care (for example, transfer to a HDU or ITU) will improve the patient's prognosis. Attending a moribund patient on the ward in extremis, or even worse in cardiac arrest, should generally be seen as a failure of previous management. Mortality increases with illness severity and the outcome after cardiac arrest in hospitalized patients is extremely poor, with less than 20% patients surviving to hospital discharge.

Although there are exceptions (such as acute massive pulmonary embolism in a post-operative patient or ventricular fibrillation cardiac arrest post-myocardial infarction), critical life-threatening illness tends to develop gradually over hours or days. Although the presenting illness often involves only one organ system, the lack of appropriate management may result in

Clinical Anaesthesia Lecture Notes, Fourth Edition. Carl Gwinnutt and Matthew Gwinnutt.
© 2012 John Wiley & Sons, Ltd. Published 2012 by John Wiley & Sons, Ltd.

multiple organ systems becoming involved and ultimately one or more organs may fail as the patient's physiological compensatory mechanisms become exhausted.

In an ideal world, the doctor attending an acutely ill patient would be a senior, experienced clinician who would expertly make a rapid assessment of the patient, initiate emergency treatment, carry out a more detailed assessment, order appropriate investigations and finally arrive at a likely clinical diagnosis and initiate definitive treatment. In the real world this is usually not the case. Routine procedure for the ward nurse concerned about a patient's condition will be to contact the most junior member of the medical team, often a Foundation Year One doctor. The reason for the call may have been that the patient's Early Warning Score (EWS – see later) has exceeded a trigger threshold. However, the nurse may also be more specific in stating that she is worried about the patient's breathing, low blood pressure, low urine output, and so on. The inexperienced clinician will need to rely on a systematic process of clinical assessment to identify which organ systems are dysfunctional or failing, what the likely diagnosis is (or differential diagnoses are) and therefore what initial management is most appropriate.

Although ultimately there is no substitute for experience, a diverse range of courses are available, which aim to 'short-circuit' the knowledge and experience gap. These courses provide intensive, often didactic, teaching by faculties of experienced multidisciplinary clinicians, including doctors from different specialties and nurses. Examples include:

- *Acute Life-threatening Event Recognition and Treatment (ALERT):* the recognition and management of patients in the early stages of developing critical illness.
- *Acute Illness Management (AIM):* the recognition and management of patients in the early stages of developing critical illness.
- *Care of the Critically Ill Surgical Patient (CCrISP):* the management of critically ill surgical patients.
- *Advanced Life Support (ALS):* the prevention and management of cardiorespiratory arrest.
- *Advanced Trauma Life Support (ATLS), European Trauma Course (ETC):* the management of major life-threatening trauma.
- *Advanced Paediatric Life Support (APLS):* the recognition and management of the sick child.

- *Situation Background Assessment Recommendation (SBAR):* communication during critical situations.

Attendance at an ALS course is mandatory for Foundation doctors (as is successfully passing the course!) and attending at least one of the courses aimed at recognizing and managing acutely ill patients cannot be recommended highly enough.

Clinical scoring systems (track and trigger systems)

In order to treat acute illness or the deterioration in a patient's condition, it first has to be recognized, often by the ward nurse in response to routine clinical observations. In the 1990s formal clinical scoring systems, often termed Early Warning Scoring Systems (EWS), were introduced to facilitate the process of assessing illness severity, 'flagging up' patients for urgent medical assessment and monitoring response to treatment. In 2007 the National Institute for Health and Clinical Excellence (NICE) published its recommendation that 'Physiological track and trigger systems should be used to monitor all adult patients in acute hospital settings.'

All EWS systems are based on the premise that acute physiological deterioration precedes the development of life-threatening acute illness and cardiorespiratory arrest. Simple observations relating to the physiological and clinical status of the patient that can be performed at the bedside on a general ward are recorded and scores are allotted for each observation based on reference to a scoring table (Table 8.1). NICE recommends that the minimum dataset should include:

- heart rate;
- respiratory rate;
- systolic blood pressure;
- level of consciousness;
- temperature;
- peripheral oxygen saturation.

Urine output is often also included. Another subjective category is sometimes added to include any patient about whom there are serious concerns, independent of the objective scoring assessment. The importance of this latter point cannot

Table 8.1 An early warning scoring system (from Prytherch DR *et al. Resuscitation* 2010; 81: 932–7)

Score	3	2	1	0	1	2	3
Pulse (/min)		≤ 40	41–50	51–90	91–110	111–130	≥ 131
Respiratory rate (/min)	≤ 8		9–11	12–20		21–24	> 25
Temperature (°C)	≤ 35.0		35.1–36.0	36.1–38.0	38.1–39.0	≤ 39.1	
Systolic BP (mmHg)	≤ 90	91–100	101–110	111–249	≥ 250		
Oxygen saturation (%)	≤ 91	92–93	94–95	≥ 96			
Inspired oxygen				Air			Any oxygen therapy
AVPU				Alert (A)			Voice (V) Pain (P) Unresponsive (U)

be overemphasized, particularly when the concern is voiced by an experienced nurse who 'doesn't like the look of' a particular patient. Although not a simple bedside observation, measurement of serum lactate concentration can provide valuable additional information (see below). The individual scores derived from each variable are aggregated and trigger thresholds are set that mandate action (for example, the ward nurse must contact the Foundation doctor who must attend the patient within a specified time frame). NICE recommends a graded response dependent on whether the aggregated score is low, medium or high:

- low score – increased frequency of observations and nurse in charge notified;
- medium score – urgent call to patient's primary medical team;
- high score – emergency call to medical emergency team/critical care outreach team (see below).

The main advantages of such scoring systems are:

- simplicity, with the need for only the basic monitoring equipment, normally present on any acute hospital ward;
- reproducibility between different observers;
- staff require a minimum of training;
- their applicability to trainee doctors, nurses (both qualified and student) and other health professionals.

Clinical scoring systems are undoubtedly useful but they cannot be relied upon to the exclusion of sound clinical judgment. They fail to identify patients who are at risk (false negatives, low sensitivity) and identify patients as being at risk when they are not (false positives, low specificity).

Critical care outreach teams

Outreach teams have been established in many hospitals to respond either to a patient with a high EWS or to assist the medical team currently managing a patient who is not responding to treatment. Outreach teams are usually multidisciplinary, although their precise makeup will vary from hospital to hospital. The team leader should be trained in the management of critically ill patients and ideally be either an experienced critical care doctor or critical care nurse practitioner. The aims of the outreach team are summarized in Table 8.2.

Receiving a call

When called to assess an acutely ill patient you may not have seen him/her previously and may have no prior knowledge of his/her medical history. Therefore, when answering a call to assess a sick patient, it is very helpful to obtain some information over the phone so that you can be thinking about possible causes and treatment as you make your way to the ward. An experienced referrer may provide a concise summary of the patient's recent history and current condition, including EWS score. However, if insufficient

---

Table 8.2 **Aims of the outreach team**

- Early identification of patients with actual or potential critical illness
- Appropriate early intervention, which may prevent deterioration and avert the need for admission to HDU or ITU
- Liaison with the HDU and ITU
- Facilitate early admission to HDU and ITU when necessary
- Identification of patients for whom HDU or ITU care is deemed inappropriate
- Appropriate early designation of patients as 'do not attempt resuscitation' in the event of cardiorespiratory arrest (DNAR order)
- To assist ward nurses in the management of patients with actual or potential critical illness
- Education and training of trainee doctors, nurses and medical students
- Promote continuity of care following step-down of patients to the ward from HDU and ITU.

---

information is volunteered you should ask a few pertinent questions:

- How old is the patient?
- When was the patient admitted to hospital?
- What is the working diagnosis?
- Is the patient conscious and, if so, what is the patient complaining of?
- How quickly has the patient deteriorated?
- What are the patient's latest vital signs – respiratory rate, heart rate, blood pressure, temperature, oxygen saturation?
- Does the patient have a 'do not attempt resuscitation' (DNAR) order?

The principles of assessment

When assessing and managing acutely ill patients, irrespective of the severity of their conditions, the initial aim must be to make the patient safe rather than to determine a precise diagnosis. Many clinical crises can be managed initially by prompt recognition and correction of a modest number of common abnormalities using simple therapies (for example, oxygen and fluids).

It is logical for all members of the healthcare team to use the same systematic approach to assess and treat the 'at risk' or acutely ill patient incorporating the following:

- primary assessment and resuscitation using the 'ABCDE' approach;
- start simple bedside monitoring;
- once immediate life-threatening conditions have been treated, secondary assessment of the patient using all available information – history, examination, investigations;

- analysis of all the information available and making a diagnosis or a list of differential diagnoses;
- a definitive management or care plan including referral to a senior colleague if you have any doubts about your ability to manage the situation safely;
- good record keeping.

> **KEY POINTS**
>
> - The aim of initial interventions is to keep the patient alive and produce some clinical improvement, so that definitive treatment may be initiated.
> - Always correct life-threatening abnormalities before moving on to the next stage of the assessment.
> - Resuscitation measures (oxygen, fluids etc.) often take a few minutes to have an effect.
> - Call for help early. At every stage of the patient assessment, consider 'do I need help?'

Once immediately life-threatening conditions have been identified and treated following your primary assessment, undertake a full secondary assessment. Reassess the patient regularly and after every intervention to determine the impact of treatment and to detect any deterioration. Do not try to do everything yourself; use all members of the multidisciplinary team, they are there to help you. To do this you must communicate effectively with everyone: staff, patient, and relatives.

There may be several interventions happening at the same time, particularly if the patient is in a peri-arrest situation; always ensure your own safety and that of the patient:

- take note of environmental hazards such as electricity and fluid spillage;

- dispose of needles and other sharps into 'sharps bins';
- protect yourself by taking universal precautions – aprons, gloves, and masks will reduce the risk of contamination from secretions, blood, and so forth.

Hygiene has an important impact on patient outcome, therefore, despite all the pressures:

- always wash your hands before and after patient contact;
- adopt an aseptic no-touch technique (ANTT) for invasive procedures.

Initial approach to the patient

Ask the patient a simple question, such as 'How are you?' A normal verbal response immediately informs you that the patient:

- has a patent airway;
- is breathing;
- has brain perfusion with oxygenated blood.

If the patient can only speak in short sentences, suspect severe respiratory distress. Failure to respond to the question is likely to suggest serious illness and you should immediately assess the patient for signs of life whilst keeping the airway open. If the patient has no signs of life, follow the current guidelines for in-hospital resuscitation (see below).

The next step is to commence an ABCDE assessment of the patient. While you are doing this, ask an assistant to attach the following as soon as is safely possible:

- pulse oximeter;
- ECG monitor;
- non-invasive blood pressure monitor.

The ABCDE system is as follows:

A is for AIRWAY.
B is for BREATHING.
C is for CIRCULATION.
D is for DISABILITY (CNS function).
E is for EXPOSURE (permitting full patient examination).

The assessment and consequent actions are prioritized in this order because, generally, airway obstruction kills faster than breathing disorders, which in turn kill faster than blood loss or cardiac dysfunction. Each part of the assessment system follows a similar pattern; the simultaneous identification and treatment of potentially life-threatening conditions.

Most abnormalities will be detected using simple clinical examination techniques based on a look–feel–listen approach. The order of the various components of the look–feel–listen approach will vary depending on the body system being examined.

Primary assessment and resuscitation

Airway assessment (A)

The aim is to identify and treat airway obstruction if present. Always treat airway obstruction as a medical emergency and obtain expert help immediately. Untreated, it leads to a lowered PaO_2, risks hypoxic damage to tissues (such as brain, kidneys and heart) and will cause cardiac arrest and death. In a critically ill patient, airway obstruction is frequently due to a depressed conscious level but there are other causes (Table 8.3). The converse is also true; if the patient is talking to you then the airway is likely to be clear.

> **KEY POINTS**
>
> - Impaired conscious level, for example due to cerebral hypoxia, drugs or acute brain injury, is the commonest cause of airway obstruction on general hospital wards.
> - Noisy breathing always indicates obstruction; silence may mean apnoea.

Look, listen and feel for the signs of airway obstruction. This is best accomplished by positioning your ear close to the patient's nose and mouth whilst looking down across the chest.

Look for chest movement:

- Paradoxical chest and abdominal movements ('see-saw' respirations).
- Use of the accessory muscles of respiration (for example sternomastoid and muscles of the neck, back, and shoulder girdle).

NOTE: central cyanosis is a late sign of airway obstruction.

Table 8.3 Causes of acute upper airway obstruction

- Depressed conscious level
- Secretions, blood, vomit
- Foreign body
- Upper airway swelling
- Upper airway tumour
- External compression of the airway
- Blocked tracheostomy
- Trauma

Listen for sounds of air movement and any associated abnormal noises:

- Complete airway obstruction is silent.
- Partial airway obstruction is noisy.
- Silence indicates either complete airway obstruction in the presence of the patient's obvious efforts to breathe or apnoea (respiratory arrest).

Certain noises assist in localizing the level of the obstruction (Table 8.4).

Feel for expired air:

- Place your hand or side of face immediately in front of the patient's mouth. This will help confirm the presence or absence of airflow and give an indication of the tidal volume.

If there are signs of obstruction, call for expert help immediately and move rapidly to using simple methods of airway clearance: a visual inspection

Table 8.4 The characteristics of airway noises assist in localizing the level of airway obstruction

Sound	Cause
• Gurgling	• Liquid in the mouth or upper airway
• Snoring	• Partial obstruction of the pharynx, usually by the tongue
• Crowing	• Laryngeal spasm
• Inspiratory stridor	• Obstruction above or at the level of the larynx
• Expiratory wheeze	• Airway collapse during expiration (e.g. asthma)
• Rattling	• Secretions in the airways

for evidence of obvious upper airway obstruction due to foreign body (for example blood, secretions, food bolus, vomit) and careful airway suction only as far as you can see using a rigid wide bore suction catheter (for example, Yankauer); head tilt and chin lift (Fig. 4.3); insertion of an oropharyngeal or naso-pharyngeal airway (see Chapter 2). If these measures fail, tracheal intubation may be required, but should only be attempted by experienced staff. In most situations, intubation will require the use of hypnotic and neuromuscular blocking drugs and an anaesthetist.

Once you are certain that the patient has a satisfactory airway, give oxygen initially at high flow (15 L/min) using a mask with an oxygen reservoir (Fig. 7.4), and move on rapidly to assess breathing. This applies to all patients who are breathless or who exhibit other signs of acute illness, including patients with COPD. Hypoxia kills quickly; hypercapnia kills much more slowly. Reassess the patient and titrate the inspired oxygen to produce an acceptable SpO_2 or PaO_2 (see below).

Assess breathing (B)

The aim is to assess adequacy of breathing and to diagnose and treat immediately life-threatening conditions such as severe bronchospasm, severe pneumonia, acute exacerbation of COPD, acute pulmonary oedema and tension pneumothorax. If untreated, inadequate breathing will lead to hypoxaemia and may also cause hypercapnia (Figs. 7.1 and 7.2), which can eventually lead to unconsciousness. There are many causes of disordered or inadequate breathing (see Table 8.5). The 'look, listen and feel' approach is used again.

Look for the signs of abnormal breathing:

- Use of the accessory muscles of respiration, tracheal tug, abdominal breathing, sweating, central cyanosis.
- Abnormal respiratory rate; normal is between 12 and 20 breaths/min. A rapid rate is an early sign of severe acute illness and should be regarded as a warning that the patient may suddenly deteriorate. An abnormally low rate suggests a CNS problem.
- Depth of each breath.
- Pattern (rhythm) of breathing.
- Symmetry of movement of the two sides of the chest.

Table 8.5 Causes of breathing problems

Primary lung dysfunction	Secondary causes
Acute • Acute asthma • Pneumonia • Pneumothorax • Acute exacerbation of COPD • Exhaustion • Haemothorax • Pulmonary contusion **Chronic** • Emphysema • Pulmonary fibrosis • Tumours • Bronchiectasis • Cystic fibrosis • Tuberculosis • Diffuse parenchymal lung disease	**Respiratory** • Airway obstruction • ARDS • Aspiration **Cardiovascular** • Heart failure • Pulmonary embolism • Cardiac tamponade **Neuromuscular problems** • Guillain–Barré syndrome • Myasthenia gravis • High spinal cord injury • Exhaustion **CNS depression** • Drugs • Head injury • Meningitis/encephalitis • Cerebral haemorrhage • Cerebral tumour • Cerebral hypoxia **Diaphragmatic splinting** • Morbidly obese patients • Abdominal pain • Abdominal distension

Also look for:

- Chest deformity, as this may impair the ability to breathe normally.
- Raised JVP (which may signify acute severe asthma or a tension pneumothorax).
- Chest drains – are they patent, below the level of the chest and swinging/draining?
- Abdominal distension, as this may exacerbate respiratory distress by limiting diaphragmatic movement.

Listen for signs of respiratory disease:

- Place your ear close to the patient's face if necessary. Rattling or gurgling airway noises indicate the presence of airway secretions, often due to the inability of the patient to cough sufficiently or to take a deep breath. Inspiratory noisy breathing (stridor) suggests partial, but significant, airway obstruction.
- Auscultate the chest, placing the stethoscope in all areas of the chest, both front and back and assess the quality of the breath sounds:
  - high-pitched expiratory noisy breathing (wheeze) suggests bronchospasm;
  - bronchial breathing suggests lung consolidation;
  - absent or reduced sounds suggest the presence of a pneumothorax or pleural effusion;
  - crackles – if fine they suggest pulmonary oedema or pulmonary fibrosis; coarse suggest retained secretions.

Feel the chest for:

- The position of the trachea in the suprasternal notch. Deviation to one side indicates mediastinal shift (for example, tension pneumothorax or massive pleural effusion).
- Equality of expansion – reduced on the side of a pneumothorax or pleural effusion.
- Surgical emphysema or crepitus – assume that this indicates a pneumothorax until proven otherwise.
- Percussion: hyper-resonance suggests a pneumothorax; dullness suggests consolidation or pleural fluid.

A pulse oximeter should be attached to the patient as soon as possible. This provides invaluable information on the net result of the patient's respiratory effort in oxygenating blood as it flows through the lungs. In most patients, the target SpO_2 should be 94–98%. Initially high-flow oxygen at 15 L/min using a mask with attached reservoir bag should be given; the inspired oxygen may be reduced later according to the patient's response. In *some* patients suffering from *severe* COPD who are dependent on a hypoxic drive for their breathing (Type II respiratory failure, chronic hypoxaemia and hypercapnia), high concentrations of oxygen may abolish their respiratory drive. Limiting the inspired oxygen concentration may be warranted if there is reasonable suspicion that the patient may have chronic type II respiratory failure. Nevertheless, this latter group of patients remains at risk of end-organ damage, cardiac arrest, or death if their blood oxygen tensions are allowed to fall too low. In this group, titrate oxygen therapy to an initial SpO_2 of 88–92%.

If possible, an arterial blood gas sample should be obtained for urgent analysis provided this does not delay moving rapidly onto assessment of the circulation. This will provide information on:

- Oxygenation, PaO_2: as a 'rule of thumb' a numerical difference between the PaO_2 (kPa) and inspired oxygen concentration (%) of more than 10 implies a defect in oxygen uptake.
- Ventilation, $PaCO_2$: hypercapnia (increased $PaCO_2$) is the result of inadequate alveolar ventilation; hypocapnia, excessive ventilation.
- Metabolism, pH, base excess: acutely ill patients usually have a metabolic acidosis (decreased pH, negative base excess) in proportion to the severity of illness. An acidosis may also be seen in diabetic ketoacidosis, or in surgical patients who lose bicarbonate via the gastrointestinal tract (for example, diarrhoea, fistulae).
- Many modern blood gas analysers will also measure electrolytes and lactate. An increase in the latter implies significant impairment of tissue oxygenation, even though the PaO_2 may be normal. This signifies a problem with oxygen delivery to the tissues and acute circulatory shock.

Any life-threatening respiratory problem should be treated as soon as it is identified. If the patient's breathing is dangerously inadequate or if the patient is apnoeic, ventilation must be assisted or controlled using a bag-valve-mask with reservoir attached to high-flow oxygen, 15 L/min, whilst calling urgently for expert help. The addition of a reservoir allows oxygen concentrations close to 100% to be given. For treatment of specific conditions see below.

🔑 **KEY POINTS**

- A pulse oximeter does not measure $PaCO_2$ and, therefore, gives no indication of the adequacy of a patient's ventilation.
- Hypoxaemic patients tend to hyperventilate, with a resultant low $PaCO_2$.
- If a patient is receiving oxygen therapy, the SpO_2 may be normal, despite inadequate ventilation.
- A normal PaO_2 (12–14 kPa) whilst breathing 100% oxygen ($FiO_2 \sim 1.0$) is not normal.

Assess the circulation (C)

The aim is to assess the patient's haemodynamic status and to recognize and treat circulatory shock, whatever the cause. Shock is inadequate perfusion of the vital organs with oxygenated blood and if untreated will lead to ischaemic damage to the vital organs and organ failure. In many surgical and medical emergencies, the cause of shock is hypovolaemia. Major haemorrhage (overt or hidden) should be assumed until proven otherwise in patients who develop shock in the early postoperative period. Respiratory pathology, such as a tension pneumothorax, can also compromise a patient's circulatory state, but should have been detected already and treated if the above system has been followed. The 'look, listen and feel' approach is used again.

Look for:

- The colour of the hands and digits; are they cyanosed, pale, or mottled, indicating poor peripheral perfusion?
- Fullness of the peripheral veins. Are they underfilled or collapsed, signifying hypovolaemia?
- The central veins. Are they collapsed, signifying hypovolaemia, or engorged signifying acute left ventricular failure, cardiac tamponade, tension pneumothorax or acute severe asthma?
- Other signs of inadequate cardiac output, such as reduced level of consciousness, oliguria (urine volume < 0.5 mL/kg/h).
- Obvious signs of blood or ECF loss; bleeding, nasogastric or other drain loss.

NOTE: empty drains do not exclude active bleeding. Haemorrhage may be concealed (for example, intrathoracic, intraperitoneal, pelvic, or into the gut).

Listen for:

- Added heart sounds. Third and fourth heart sounds are heard in diastole and result in a triple rhythm – a gallop rhythm. A third heart sound (early diastole) is indicative of heart failure; a fourth heart sound (late diastole) is also indicative of stiff, poorly functioning left ventricle.
- A heart murmur, usually indicative of valvular heart disease.
- A pericardial rub, indicative of pericarditis.
- Very quiet heart sounds, these may be heard in severe emphysema and pericardial effusion.

Feel for:

- Limb temperature by feeling the patient's hands and feet. Are they warm, or cool suggesting poor perfusion?
- A central pulse (usually the carotid artery) and compare with a peripheral pulse (usually the radial artery). Assess for:
  - rate;
  - rhythm/regularity;
  - volume;
  - character.

A rapid, weak, low-volume pulse suggests a poor cardiac output. A bounding pulse may indicate sepsis. Measure the patient's blood pressure. The causes of hypotension are listed in Table 8.6.

Finally, measure the capillary refill time (CRT) both centrally and peripherally. Apply firm pressure to a finger tip or toe for 5 s (at heart level or just above) and release: the capillaries should refill (colour returns to the compressed area) in <2 s. Capillary refill time may be affected by the environmental temperature. Repeat the procedure over the sternum.

Heart rate and blood pressure must be placed in context; an elderly patient with poor myocardial reserve may be in extremis with a heart rate of 60/min and blood pressure of 95/60 mmHg, but the same values will be well tolerated or even normal for a fit young adult. Ultimately, definitive treatment of shock will be determined by the cause, the most common being hypovolaemia, sepsis and cardiac failure. These are covered below.

> **🔑 KEY POINTS**
>
> - Resting heart rate is normally lower than systolic blood pressure.
> - In some patients, for example those with gastro-intestinal or intra-abdominal haemorrhage, immediate surgery may be required as the only effective form of resuscitation.
> - Patients with cardiac failure do just as badly if the heart is underfilled as if it is overfilled and so may benefit from intravenous fluids.

Assessing neurological state – disability (D)

The aim is to assess the patient's conscious level, identify any impairment and treat the cause if possible. Common causes of unconsciousness are shown in Table 8.7. Hypoxaemia, hypercapnia, or cerebral hypoperfusion should have been detected and treated at an earlier stage of the ABCDE assessment.

Examine the pupils for size and reactivity to light:

- Pinpoint pupils, reactive: opioids, pontine lesion.
- Mid-sized, fixed: lesion in the midbrain.

Table 8.6 Causes of systemic hypotension

- Absolute hypovolaemia
  - Dehydration; inadequate input, excessive output
  - Haemorrhage
  - Burns
- Relative hypovolaemia
  - Sepsis
  - Anaphylaxis
  - Spinal cord injury
  - Epidural/spinal anaesthesia
- Cardiogenic
  - Acute myocardial infarction
  - Arrhythmia
  - Severe valvular heart disease
  - Cardiac tamponade
- Obstructive
  - Massive pulmonary embolus
  - Tension pneumothorax
- Drug overdose – e.g. antihypertensives

Table 8.7 Common causes of a decreased conscious level

- Hypoxaemia
- Hypotension
- Hypercapnia
- Hypoglycaemia
- Hyponatraemia
- Drugs (e.g., sedatives, opiates, overdoses)
- Seizures
- Head injury
- Intracranial haemorrhage
- Cerebral infarction
- Intracranial infection
- Cerebral neoplasm
- Hypothermia
- Hyperthermia
- Hypothyroidism
- Hepatic encephalopathy

- Dilated, fixed: severe global ischaemia or hypoxia (for example, post-cardiac arrest), hypoglycaemia, brainstem lesion, post-seizure, drug effects (for example, atropine, adrenaline, overdose of tricyclic antidepressant).
- Unilateral dilatation, fixed: expanding intracranial haematoma causing uncal herniation, lesion of third (occulomotor) cranial nerve.

Other important checks:

- Assess the patient's conscious level using the GCS (Table 8.8) and record the best response.
- Immediately check the patient's glucose using a rapid bedside Point of Care Testing (POCT) blood analyser to exclude severe hypoglycaemia and send blood urgently for more accurate laboratory estimation.
- Check the patient's drug chart for reversible drug-induced causes of depressed consciousness.
- Consider the possibility of acute CNS infection, intracranial haemorrhage or cerebral infarct.
- Status epilepticus should be obvious and treated as described below.

Table 8.8 The Glasgow Coma Scale

Assessment and response	Score
Eye opening	
• Spontaneous	4
• To speech	3
• To pain	2
• None	1
Verbal response	
• Orientated	5
• Confused	4
• Inappropriate words	3
• Incomprehensible sounds	2
• None	1
Best motor response	
• Obeys commands	6
• Localizes to pain	5
• Withdraws from pain	4
• Abnormal flexion to pain	3
• Extension to pain	2
• None	1

Highest achievable score is 15; the lowest score is 3. Coma is defined as a score of 8 or less; patients have no eye-opening (1), no verbalization (2), do not obey commands (5).

🔑 KEY POINTS

- Patients who are in coma (GCS < 9) are at risk of airway obstruction when supine and airway reflexes may be insufficient to prevent aspiration of secretions, vomit or blood. Nurse in the recovery position and summon expert help to secure their airway.
- If there is a risk of co-existing cervical spine pathology, for example a fracture, nurse the patient supine maintaining a patent airway. This mandates the constant presence of a nurse or doctor.
- Don't Ever Forget Glucose (DEFG) in any patient with acute deterioration in conscious level.

Exposure/examination (E)

The aim is to allow a full, head-to-toe, back and front examination of the patient. To allow this, full exposure of the body is necessary, carried out in a way that respects the dignity of the patient and prevents heat loss. Initially, the examination should be focused on the area of the body most likely to be causing the patient's condition; for example, for a patient presenting with shock following a laparotomy, this would be the abdomen. If this step is omitted, vital information regarding the aetiology of the patient's condition may be missed, such as the presence of a purpuric rash signifying meningococcal septicaemia, or a knife stab wound in the back of the chest.

What to do next?

The aim so far has been to assess the patient, treat immediately life-threatening problems, and produce some clinical improvement, to enable a diagnosis to be made and definitive treatment initiated. Even if the patient's vital signs are still outside the normal range, they should be moving in a direction of improvement. If not, it is essential to summon senior help and, while waiting for this to arrive, reassess the patient using the ABCDE approach to try and identify the cause.

Once things are improving, gather more information about the patient:

- Take a full history from the patient, staff, relatives or the hospital notes. Comorbid conditions (such as ischaemic heart disease, COPD) can have a significant impact upon a patient's response to critical illness and must not be overlooked.
- If not already done, perform a full examination of the patient, using a traditional clinical examination format.
- Review the patient's notes and charts. Assimilate the data on charts by systematic analysis. Study both absolute values of vital signs and their trends.
- Check that important routine medications are prescribed and being administered. Look for potential interactions.
- Review the results of all laboratory and radiological investigations.

Consider if you have a credible diagnosis that accounts for the patient's condition and recent deterioration:

- if yes, consider the definitive treatment of the patient's underlying condition;
- if no, reassess the patient in case you have missed something important. Involve senior colleagues.

Consider which level of care is required by the patient (for example, ward, HDU, ITU). This may be dictated by your hospital's policies. Make complete entries in the patient's notes of your findings, assessment, and treatment. Record the patient's response to therapy. Ensure that your entry in the notes is legible, signed, dated, and timed.

Communicating information about patient deterioration

Although the systems outlined above will allow the recognition, initial assessment, and treatment of the acutely ill patient, on the majority of occasions more senior help will be required to manage the problem safely and effectively. The key to achieving this is good communication at all levels:

- Know why you are calling before picking up the phone.
- Before making the call, gather all the useful information together.

- Do you want a more senior colleague to assess the patient?
- Are you calling for advice?
- Do you think the patient needs an operation, transfer to a critical care area, CT scan etc?
- Be assertive when communicating, avoid aggression, and be honest. 'I am unsure of what to do next' or 'I am worried that I am missing something' are likely to assist in obtaining help.
- Get the message across in the first two sentences: 'This is Dr . . . I am sorry to disturb you, but Mr Smith is deteriorating and I think that he may need an urgent operation.'

🔑 **KEY POINTS**

- Always fully expose the patient after ABCD.
- Use a system for communicating patient deterioration, e.g. RSVP or SBAR:

R – Reason for calling	S – Situation
S – Story	B – Background
V – Vital signs (plus	A – Assessment
any early warning	R – Recommendation
score)	
P – Plan	

Section 2: Management of common emergencies

Once an initial ABCDE assessment with treatment of immediately life-threatening problems has been performed, attention will need to be focused on determining the underlying problem and beginning appropriate definitive treatment. The following is intended to provide a practical approach to the important aspects of the management of some common emergencies. In most acutely ill patients, initial treatment and investigations will occur simultaneously; they have been separated below for clarity. Clearly, there will frequently be areas of overlap of symptoms and signs, for example pulmonary embolism may present with shortness of breath, chest pain, hypotension, loss of consciousness or cardiac arrest. In all acute situations get senior help early.

Acute shortness of breath

You will be called often to assess patients who are breathless (dyspnoeic). Respiratory rate is one of the key parameters in all EWS systems and is perhaps the single most sensitive indicator of a potentially life-threatening critical illness. Taking a history from the patient can be challenging if he is too breathless to speak in sentences. This is itself an indicator of an *immediately* life-threatening condition.

There are many causes of acute dyspnoea (Table 8.5). However, the differential diagnosis can be narrowed by taking into account the history, examination findings, and the results of blood tests and other investigations such as chest X-ray and 12-lead ECG. Some of the more common causes of shortness of breath are covered in more detail below.

Acute upper airway obstruction

If any patient has signs of airway obstruction *expert help should be called for immediately* (usually an anaesthetist and depending on the situation, an ENT surgeon). Common causes are shown in Table 8.3. However, while waiting for help to arrive it is possible to quickly and safely start the process of restoring a patent airway and delivering oxygen. Examine the patient for signs of upper airway obstruction.

Look for:

- distress in the patient;
- use of accessory muscles, often sat upright, flaring of the alae nasae;
- dyspnoea, rapid shallow breaths;
- see-saw or paradoxical respiratory pattern;
- drooling, not swallowing saliva;
- cyanosis.

Listen for:

- abnormal sounds, stridor, wheeze, gurgling;
- reduced or absent breath sounds;
- inability to vocalize, poor voice strength.

Feel for:

- reduced air movement at the face;
- decreased chest expansion;

- pulse rate – this is increased due to hypoxia and hypercapnia.

Other features may be apparent with obstruction due to specific causes and are covered below:

- a reduced conscious level (reduced GCS);
- swelling of the upper airway or tumour;
- external compression of the airway, for example after surgery;
- a blocked tracheostomy or laryngectomy stoma.

Reduced conscious level (reduced GCS)

This may be either the result of, or the cause of, airway obstruction. In either case, relief of the obstruction is the first step in management.

1 Carry out a visual inspection of the airway and suction of any oral/oro-pharyngeal debris.
2 Open the airway using simple manoeuvres such as head tilt, chin lift, and jaw thrust and check for any spontaneous breathing.
3 If breathing is inadequate or absent, use a self-inflating bag with reservoir and face mask attached to 15 L/min oxygen to assist ventilation.
4 Ventilate by achieving a good seal around the patient's nose and mouth with the facemask and gentle squeezing of the self-inflating bag. This may require a two-person technique.
5 If these basic manoeuvres are inadequate use a simple airway adjunct, for example using naso- or oropharyngeal airways. If you are trained and it is available, use a supraglottic airway device (for example, LMA, i-gel).
6 Establish basic monitoring including a pulse oximeter, non-invasive blood pressure, and ECG (this can be monitored via defibrillator pads).
7 Once a patent airway and oxygenation is established, check for cardiac output. If it is absent, follow the advanced life-support algorithm for cardiac arrest (see below).
8 A suitably trained member of staff may decide that tracheal intubation is needed.

Once the patient has been stabilized with an adequate airway and ventilation and is haemodynamically stable, the next step is to identify the reason for the reduced GCS (see below).

Upper airway swelling/tumour

Swelling of the upper airway may result from infection, allergic reactions, smoke inhalation or ingestion of caustic liquids. Tumours of the pharynx and larynx may also lead to upper airway obstruction. The cause can often be elicited from an accurate history either from the patient, if they are still able to talk, from an accompanying person or the patient's medical notes. Specific findings may include:

- inability to visualize the posterior wall of the oropharynx due to swelling;
- soot in the nares and mouth along with singed facial hair in burns:
  - do not force the patient to lie down – gravity may be helping maintain the airway;

Start treatment:

- Give high-flow oxygen via facemask with reservoir.
- Establish basic monitoring including a pulse oximeter, non-invasive blood pressure, and ECG (this can be monitored via defibrillator pads).
- If an inflammatory cause is suspected:
  - start treatment with nebulized adrenaline (5 mL 1:1000) in oxygen;
  - establish IV access and give 8 mg dexamethasone IV.
- When there is a 'threatened airway':
  - nasendoscopy by an experienced operator may provide information about the cause and potential difficulties with intubation;
  - if safe, transfer the patient to either a critical care area or operating theatre;
  - an experienced doctor may use 'Heliox', a mixture of oxygen and helium (this reduces the work of breathing), but this will reduce the inspired oxygen concentration.
- If the airway obstructs completely, depending on the skills available:
  - attempt oxygenation via face mask and self-inflating bag;
  - insert a supraglottic airway, attempt ventilation;
  - direct laryngoscopy, attempt tracheal intubation with small diameter (6 mm) tube;
  - perform a surgical airway.
- Once oxygenation is established, transfer to the operating theatre for a definitive airway.

External compression after surgery

There are a number of operations that involve surgical access to, and dissection in, the anterior triangle of the neck – for example thyroidectomy,

parathyroidectomy, carotid endarterectomy and cervical disc surgery. The commonest cause of obstruction is development of a haematoma, causing compression of the larynx, displacement of the trachea, and laryngeal mucosal engorgement and oedema, all of which lead to airway compromise. More rarely, surgery may inadvertently damage the recurrent laryngeal nerve lying between the trachea and larynx anteriorly, and the oesophagus posteriorly. Airway compromise usually only follows bilateral damage. Specific findings may include:

- neck swelling;
- bleeding from the wound;
- blocked surgical drain.

Start treatment:

- Give high-flow oxygen and establish basic monitoring.
- Inform the surgical team as the patient will probably need to be returned to theatre.
- Consider nebulized adrenaline and steroids as described above to reduce any oedema.
- If the neck is obviously swollen, open the surgical incision to allow evacuation of the haematoma and release of the pressure upon the airway.
- Attempt to support ventilation using a facemask and self-inflating bag with 100% oxygen.
- If evacuation of the haematoma does not relieve the obstruction (because of severe laryngeal oedema):
  - direct laryngoscopy by an experienced anaesthetist may allow tracheal intubation;
  - equipment for a surgical airway must be immediately available.

In the case of recurrent laryngeal nerve injury bag-valve-mask ventilation should be performed initially. Tracheal intubation is usually achievable once hypnotics and a neuromuscular blocking drug have been given.

Blocked tracheostomy

Tracheostomies are performed for a variety of clinical indications including upper airway obstruction, to facilitate weaning from mechanical ventilation, to allow long-term ventilation and to provide a route to allow removal of secretions from the patient's respiratory tract. A tracheostomy can be temporary or permanent.

The patient's airway can be compromised either because the tube has become blocked or displaced. Rapid relief of the occlusion usually allows oxygenation but if the tube is displaced it may be the cause of airway obstruction. It may then be necessary to remove the tube to allow the patient to breathe via the tracheostomy track, the normal airway or a combination of both. The process for safe management of these patients is shown in Fig. 8.1.

In contrast a laryngectomy is usually performed for carcinoma of the larynx and results in permanent alteration of the patient's airway. These patients are often referred to as 'neck breathers' and rely on their tracheostomy for ventilation. Complications can occur at the time of the procedure (bleeding), after the procedure (obstruction, displacement) or long term (tracheomalacia, tracheal stenosis). Many of these patients may not have a tracheostomy tube *in situ* but may have a device to allow 'oesophageal speech'. The process for safe management of these patients is shown in Fig. 8.2.

Acute lower airway problems

Having assessed and eliminated an upper airway problem as the cause of shortness of breath (see above), consideration can be given to lower airway problems. These can either be due to primary lung dysfunction or are secondary to other conditions (Table 8.5). Examine the patient for signs and symptoms of lower airway obstruction.

Look for:

- dyspnoea;
- increased respiratory rate;
- reduced chest expansion;
- use of accessory muscles;
- abdominal breathing pattern;
- tracheal tug.

Listen for:

- rattling or gurgling noises;
- wheeze;
- abnormal breath sounds on auscultation;
- murmurs, additional heart sounds.

Feel for:

- air movement at the face;
- altered percussion note;

- position of the trachea;
- subcutaneous emphysema.

Other features may be apparent with acute lower airway problems due to specific causes and the following are covered in more detail below:

- acute severe asthma;
- pneumonia;
- pneumothorax;
- pulmonary oedema;
- pulmonary embolus.

Acute severe asthma

Although many of the above features may be present, asthma is typically associated with wheeziness. However when severe, the patient may not be wheezy because of minimal air movement into the chest – the so called 'silent chest'. Such patients may also be cyanosed and have a reduced level of consciousness. If any one of the following is present, the patient has acute severe asthma:

- severe breathlessness – unable to complete sentences in one breath;
- respiratory rate > 25/min, heart rate > 110/min;
- if measurable, peak expiratory flow (PEF) 33–50% best or predicted.

The British Thoracic Society (BTS) and Scottish Intercollegiate Guidelines Network (SIGN) have produced guidelines on the management of asthma. The following is based on the current guidelines (see useful information section).

Start treatment with:

- high flow oxygen;
- high dose nebulized beta-2 agonist, salbutamol 5 mg repeated.

Establish basic monitoring:

- pulse oximetry;
- non-invasive blood pressure;
- ECG (can be monitored via defibrillator pads).

Gain IV access:

- give steroids IV, hydrocortisone 100 mg.

If there is little or no response:

- give magnesium sulphate, 8 mmol (2 g) slowly IV;
- add nebulized ipratropium 0.5 mg;
- take an arterial blood sample for blood gas analysis.

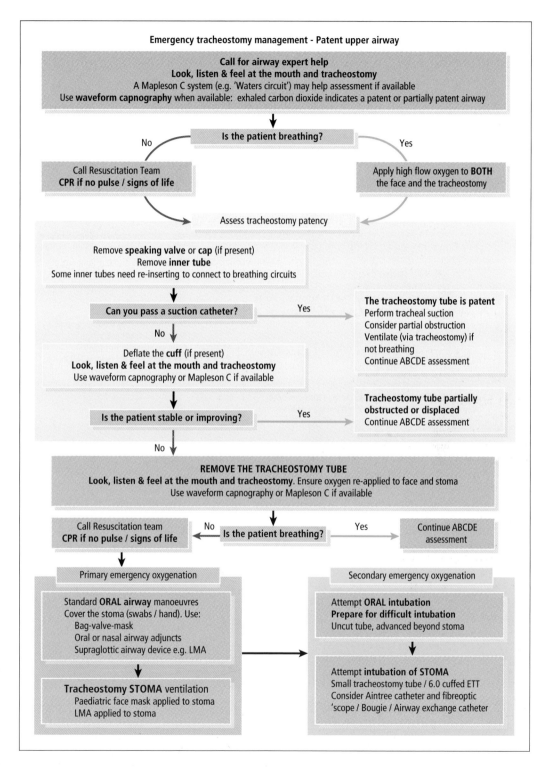

Figure 8.1 Algorithm for emergency tracheostomy management (courtesy of the National Tracheostomy Safety Project).

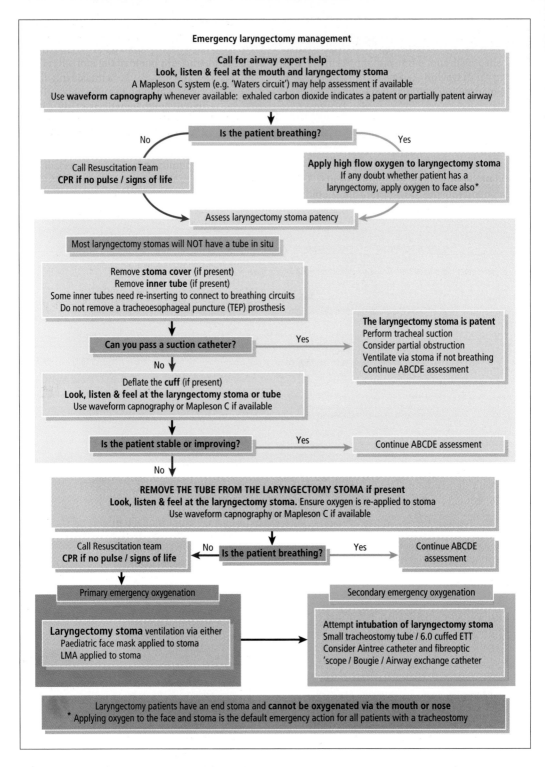

Figure 8.2 Algorithm for emergency laryngectomy management (courtesy of the National Tracheostomy Safety Project).

Refer to ITU if:

- decreasing PEF despite treatment;
- increasing hypoxia, $PaO_2 < 8\,kPa$;
- hypercapnia, $PaCO_2 > 6.0\,kPa$;
- increasing acidosis;
- exhaustion with reduced respiratory effort;
- reduced level of consciousness.

Pneumonia

Pneumonia may be the underlying reason for a patient presenting to hospital, or it may develop during a patient's stay in hospital – for example, atelectasis and sputum retention after abdominal surgery. Pneumonia may develop at any time secondary to aspiration of gastric contents, for example at induction or emergence from anaesthesia, vomiting at any time during impaired consciousness, or due to neuromuscular disorders affecting laryngeal reflexes. On this basis pneumonia is broadly classified as community-acquired pneumonia (CAP), hospital-acquired pneumonia (HAP), or aspiration pneumonia. A patient has to have been in hospital for >48 hours prior to the onset of symptoms in order to diagnose HAP. The type of pneumonia has implications for the likely causative pathogens and hence appropriate antimicrobial treatment. There are three aspects to make the diagnosis of pneumonia.

1. History

- Ask specifically about:
  - dyspnoea;
  - cough;
  - pleuritic chest pain;
  - purulent sputum;
  - high temperature, sweating;
  - malaise.

2. Examination

- Look for:
  - confusion;
  - pyrexia;
  - dyspnoea at rest, tachypnoea;
  - cyanosis, low SpO_2;
  - hypotension.
- Listen for:
  - reduced air entry and possible crackles or bronchial breathing over the affected area, increased vocal resonance, and a pleural rub.
- Feel for:
  - a tachycardia;
  - unequal chest expansion;
  - percussion – dullness over the affected area (especially if there is an associated effusion).

Start treatment:

- Oxygen via a face mask, aiming for SpO_2 94–98% (88–92% is acceptable in patients with severe COPD). If there is a large area of consolidation the SpO_2 may not improve significantly.

Obtain IV access:

- Before connecting the IV fluid, take blood for the investigations (see below).
- Start IV fluids (Hartmann's solution); give a fluid challenge if hypotensive.
- Commence IV antibiotic therapy according to local policy and likely type of pneumonia – discussion with a microbiologist may be needed.

Start physiotherapy to encourage coughing; consider analgesia for pleuritic chest pain to improve the ability to cough but use caution with the dose of opioids if given.

Establish basic monitoring and record vital signs:

- pulse oximetry, ECG;
- BP, pulse rate;
- respiratory rate;
- temperature;
- GCS.

3. Investigations

- Take blood for full blood count (FBC), urea and electrolytes (U + Es), liver function tests (LFTs), C-reactive protein (CRP) and blood cultures.
- Take an arterial blood sample for blood gas analysis and blood lactate levels. There is often hypoxia with a normal $PaCO_2$, and a metabolic acidosis if the patient is septic.
- Obtain a CXR. There may be consolidation with loss of volume of one hemi-thorax, and an associated pleural effusion.

Patients with severe pneumonia, or those with pre-existing lung disease, may not respond to initial treatment. Early consideration should be given to ITU admission when the patient shows signs of:

- Hypoxaemia, despite a high FiO_2 for example $SpO_2 < 90\%$ or $PaO_2 < 8\,kPa$.
- Tiring, becoming drowsy, $PaCO_2$ rising.
- Hypotension, not responding to fluid challenges, or a metabolic acidosis (both imply septic shock).

Pneumothorax

This may occur spontaneously (usually in young males) or due to underlying COPD, asthma, lung carcinoma or penetrating chest trauma. A small pneumothorax may be asymptomatic. Specific findings may include complaints of sudden onset, unilateral, pleuritic chest pain.

Look for:

- dyspnoea;
- unequal chest expansion;
- wounds.

Listen for:

- decreased air entry on the affected side.

Feel for:

- decreased chest expansion on the affected side;
- percussion – hyper-resonance on the affected side;
- surgical emphysema.

Start treatment with:

- High-flow oxygen via face mask with reservoir – this will help limit or reduce the size of the pneumothorax.

Establish basic monitoring:

- pulse oximeter, ECG (can be monitored via defibrillator pads);
- blood pressure, pulse rate;
- respiratory rate;
- GCS.

Gain IV access:

- start slow infusion of fluid;
- give analgesia if required.

Investigations:

- Arrange CXR:
  - if pneumothorax is >20% radiographic lung volume, aspirate air;
  - under strict asepsis and local anaesthesia, insert a 16 g needle into the chest in the second intercostal space, mid-clavicular line;
  - connect to a 50 mL syringe via a three-way tap;
  - aspirate up to 2.5 L air or until the patient starts to cough or resistance is felt.
- Repeat CXR after attempt to drain the pneumothorax.

If the pneumothorax recurs, it will need drainage via a tube thoracostomy.

Tension pneumothorax

Occasionally the volume of air in the pleural cavity increases rapidly, either because it is sucked in during inspiration, because it fails to escape during expiration, or air is forced in during positive pressure ventilation. It is most commonly associated with trauma but may occur after insertion of a CVP line if the needle accidentally punctures the pleura. The effect is a gradual increase in intrathoracic pressure, initially causing the lung to collapse followed by shift of the mediastinum, impaired venous return and cardiovascular collapse. This is an immediately life-threatening condition and unless treated urgently will cause cardiac arrest. Specific findings include:

- severe respiratory distress, markedly tachypnoeic;
- distended neck veins (only if the patient is not hypovolaemic);
- cyanosis;
- decreased movement of one hemithorax – it may appear hyperinflated and immobile;
- absent breath sounds on the affected side;
- hyper-resonance on the affected side;
- tachycardia and hypotension;
- tracheal deviation away from the affected side – usually a pre-arrest finding.

Start treatment:

- Give high flow oxygen via facemask with reservoir.
- Gain IV access, start rapid fluid bolus.
- If the patient is in extremis, insert a 14 g or 16 g needle into the chest in the second intercostal space, mid-clavicular line on the affected side. This will relieve the pressure and create a simple pneumothorax. It is a temporizing measure only.
- Alternatively, perform a thoracostomy in the fifth intercostal space, mid-axillary line, on the affected side.
- Arrange for insertion of tube thoracostomy.
- Arrange for CXR.

🔑 **KEY POINTS**

- Do not delay decompression of the chest by requesting an X-ray. Tension pneumothorax is a clinical diagnosis.

Table 8.9 Causes of pulmonary oedema

Increased trans-capillary pressure	Increased capillary permeability
• ACS	• Severe sepsis
• Severe bradycardia	• Aspiration pneumonitis
• Severe tachycardia	• Acute panceatitis
• Severe valvular heart disease	• Major trauma
• Fluid overload, e.g. iatrogenic, renal failure	• Massive blood transfusion
• Infective endocarditis/ myocarditis	• ABO blood group incompatible transfusion
• Pericardial effusion/ cardiac tamponade	• Embolism; fat or amniotic fluid
	• Burns; cutaneous or inhalational injury

Pulmonary oedema

Although a small amount of fluid normally pass from pulmonary capillaries into the interstitial space of the lungs, the alveoli of the lungs are normally 'dry' and this interstitial fluid is drained off via the lymphatic system. However, when the rate of trans-capillary fluid migration is excessive, the lymphatic system cannot accommodate it and both interstitial and alveolar oedema develops. Although the list of causes of pulmonary oedema is long (Table 8.9) pulmonary oedema is commonly associated with two conditions:

- an increase in the trans-capillary hydrostatic pressure seen in left ventricular failure (LVF);
- an increase in pulmonary capillary permeability seen in severe sepsis and acute respiratory distress syndrome (ARDS).

The following is based on treating a patient with pulmonary oedema secondary to acute LVF. When asked to see a patient, pulmonary oedema is suggested by a number of clinical findings.

Look for:

- signs of respiratory failure:
  ○ dyspnoea;
  ○ tachypnoeic;
  ○ central cyanosis or pallor;
- cough with pink, frothy sputum;
- sweating;
- distended neck veins (raised jugular venous pressure).

Listen for:

- fine, inspiratory crackles/crepitations;
- wheeze;
- the presence of additional heart sounds (gallop rhythm);
- heart murmurs.

Feel for:

- displaced apex beat;
- apical heave.

Start treatment:

- Give high-flow oxygen therapy using a face-mask and attached reservoir bag at a flow rate of 15 L/min.
- Sit the patient as upright as possible; this reduces venous return to the heart, pulmonary capillary pressure and left ventricular filling pressure.

Establish basic monitoring:

- pulse oximeter, ECG (can be monitored via defibrillator pads);
- blood pressure, pulse rate;
- respiratory rate;
- GCS.

Gain IV access:

- Give intravenous diuretics (for example, furosemide 20–100 mg in divided doses); this causes vasodilatation and reduces preload and afterload, followed by a diuresis, which further reduces preload.
- Further preload reduction can be produced by an intravenous infusion of nitrates, such as isosorbide dinitrate. The infusion is usually started at 2 mg/h and gradually increased in increments to the maximum rate possible whilst still maintaining systolic blood pressure >100 mmHg.
- Carefully titrated IV diamorphine (up to 5 mg in 1 mg aliquots); this reduces anxiety, excessive sympathetic nervous system activity and also provides further vasodilatation.

Investigations:

- CXR; may be pathognomonic of pulmonary oedema and is key to a firm diagnosis (Fig. 8.3);
- 12-lead ECG; this is essential to confirm or refute the possibility of an acute coronary syndrome (ACS) as the cause (Fig. 8.4)

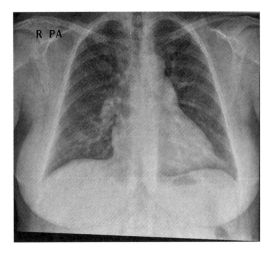

Figure 8.3 CXR showing acute pulmonary oedema.

Further measures:

- Continuous positive airway pressure (CPAP) via a facemask may be beneficial and is sometimes available on acute medical wards. It improves oxygenation by:
  - increasing the functional residual capacity (FRC), reducing the work of breathing;
  - reopens closed and under ventilated alveoli (recruitment) thereby reducing intrapulmonary shunting;
  - reduces left ventricular preload and afterload, reducing the degree of heart failure;
- If the patient does not improve with these measures, consideration should be given to treating

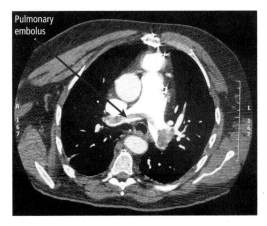

Figure 8.4 CT angiogram showing 'saddle' embolus in the pulmonary artery

with an inotrope (for example, dobutamine), particularly if hypotension is also present.
- Carefully selected patients may be transferred to the critical care unit for invasive ventilation.

Pulmonary embolism

This is a common cause of morbidity and mortality in hospitalized patients, the majority of which can be prevented through adequate risk stratification and prophylaxis as described in Chapter 1. Despite these measures, some patients will still go on to develop a pulmonary embolism (PE), which can present with collapse and PEA cardiac arrest. The probability of the patient having had a PE can be assessed using the Wells score. A numeric value is assigned to the following criteria, the greater the sum, the greater probability of a PE:

- surgery or immobilization within the previous four weeks;
- malignancy;
- previous history of DVT/pulmonary embolism;
- haemoptysis;
- tachycardia, > 100/min;
- clinical symptoms of a DVT;
- alternative diagnosis less likely than PE.

On assessment, identify specific features suggesting a PE.

Look for:

- signs of respiratory failure;
- distended neck veins;
- clinical evidence of a deep venous thrombosis (DVT).

Listen for:

- pleural rub;
- heart murmur associated with acute tricuspid regurgitation;
- additional heart sounds (gallop rhythm), widely split second heart sound.

Feel for:

- tachycardia and hypotension;
- pulsus paradoxus.

Other findings include:

- chest pain;
- haemoptysis;
- pyrexia;
- syncope;
- (specific ECG changes – see below).

Start treatment:

This will depend, to an extent, on the severity of the PE:

- All patients should initially be given oxygen therapy using a facemask and attached reservoir bag at a flow rate of 15 L/min.
- Many patients will require analgesia.
- All patients will require anticoagulation with either subcutaneous low molecular weight heparin or an intravenous infusion of unfractionated heparin until the diagnosis is confirmed/excluded and oral anticoagulation therapy established if appropriate.

In severe cases:

- Secure venous access (16 g cannula or larger); give a fluid challenge, 500 mL of warmed crystalloid or colloid. This should be repeated up to a volume of 2 L if a satisfactory response is not obtained.
- Inotropes or vasopressors may be necessary in a peri-arrest situation to support the circulation. This will require urgent advice from critical care specialists.
- Intravenous thrombolytic therapy should be initiated if there are signs of circulatory collapse, such as severe hypotension or arrhythmia, and only after other diagnoses, which would render such treatment dangerous, have been reasonably excluded.

The BTS have published guidelines on the management of suspected acute pulmonary embolism (see useful information).

Investigations:

- Chest X-ray: often unremarkable although occasionally one or both pulmonary arteries appear prominent and a peripheral wedge-shaped abnormality in one of the lung fields may be secondary to pulmonary infarction. There may be loss of the costophrenic angle due to a small effusion.
- ECG: the commonest abnormality is sinus tachycardia. Specific features suggesting right heart strain and the classical S1, Q3, T3 pattern are rarely seen, and have a low negative predictive value when absent.
- Arterial blood gas analysis will show hypoxaemia and hypocapnia in cases of significant pulmonary embolism but this is relatively non-specific.

- D-Dimer (a fibrin degradation product) assay. Almost always raised in cases of acute pulmonary embolism. Unfortunately there are other causes for increased D-Dimer. A negative result usually rules out the diagnosis.
- Imaging. Definitive diagnosis may require ventilation perfusion scan or CT pulmonary angiography (CTPA) (Fig. 8.4). Echocardiography, which can be performed at the patient's bedside, will show abnormalities of the right heart in around half of all patients with significant pulmonary embolism.

Hypotension

This is a common reason for being called to see an acutely unwell patient, particularly in the postoperative period. Blood pressure is measured in all patients routinely and is a key element in all EWS systems, but surprisingly it is not a particularly sensitive or specific indicator of the presence of a life-threatening problem unless the value is extremely high or low.

There are many causes of hypotension (Table 8.6) but, as with disturbances of other systems, the diagnosis of the cause can be determined by taking into account the history, examination findings and results of investigations. After elimination of airway and breathing problems as a cause for the hypotension, examine the patient for the following signs and symptoms.

Look for:

- evidence of impaired cerebral perfusion; conscious level:
  - orientated – good;
  - confused/agitated – bad;
  - unresponsive – worse;
- tachypnoea, dyspnoea;
- colour; pale, cyanosed, flushed;
- sweating;
- neck veins; collapsed or distended (raised jugular venous pressure).

Listen for:

- abnormal breath sounds; fine inspiratory crackles and/or (cardiac) wheeze;
- the presence of additional heart sounds (gallop rhythm) or a murmur;
- altered or absent breath sounds.

Feel for:

- pulse – rate, volume (central – for example carotid, femoral – and peripheral, for example radial, dorsalis pedis) and regularity;
- capillary refill time:
  - firm pressure applied over the sternum (central refill time) and to a digit (peripheral refill time) for 5 s to produce blanching;
  - prompt return of colour within 2 s maximum is normal;
  - delayed peripheral capillary refill suggests a low cardiac output and or perfusion pressure, delayed central capillary refill is an ominous sign;
  - unreliable in hypothermic patients;
- position of the apex beat;
- position of the trachea.

Finally, look at the patient's fluid balance chart, in particular the urine output over the previous 12 hours.

These patients are often referred to as being in 'shock'. Strictly speaking shock is defined as 'inadequate perfusion of the tissues with oxygenated blood' and although hypotension is a common feature, it may not always be present initially. Because of its common usage, the following types of shock are covered in more detail below:

- hypovolaemic shock;
- septic shock;
- cardiogenic shock.

Anaphylaxis as a cause of shock is covered in Chapter 6.

Hypovolaemic shock

Common causes of hypovolaemia include bleeding (external or concealed), excessive losses from the gastrointestinal tract (for example, diarrhoea, vomiting, fistula loss), excessive third-space losses after major tissue trauma and the relative hypovolaemia that occurs with epidural anaesthesia. The latter two causes are covered in Chapter 7.

Specific findings in hypovolaemia are manifestations of the increase in sympathetic outflow:

- vasoconstriction; causing pallor, peripheral cyanosis, cold extremities, delayed capillary refill;
- empty peripheral veins;
- tachycardia;
- sweating;

- narrowing of the pulse pressure;
- oliguria.

In the post-surgery patient, ongoing haemorrhage will be suggested by:

- a large volume of blood in the surgical drains, or from a wound;
- a distending abdomen;
- wound swelling.

Start treatment:

- All patients should be given oxygen via a face-mask and reservoir at a flow rate of 15 L/min.
- In all cases, obtain large bore venous access (14 or 16 g cannula). The antecubital fossa is often the best site for the largest vein. In severe hypovolaemia two cannulae should be inserted, one on either side. Before connecting the IV fluid, take blood for the investigations (see below):
  - give a rapid fluid challenge (over 5–10 min);
  - 500 mL of warmed crystalloid solution (for example, 0.9% saline or Hartmann's solution), if the patient's SBP is >100 mmHg;
  - 1000 mL of warmed crystalloid solution, if the patient's SBP is <100 mmHg;
  - 250 mL of warmed crystalloid solution, if the patient has pre-existing cardiac failure.

The choice of fluid (crystalloid versus colloid) is not as important as the fact that some fluid is being given. Avoid dextrose-containing fluids, they rapidly distribute throughout the total body water and have minimal intravascular effect. In addition, they cause hyperglycaemia, which is associated with increased mortality in critically ill patients.

- Reassess the pulse rate and blood pressure regularly (every 5 min), watching for signs of improvement; decreased pulse rate, increased blood pressure, improved level of consciousness. If not already done, consider inserting a urinary catheter. A urine output of 0.5–1.0 mL/kg/h suggests adequate vital organ perfusion.
- Repeat the fluid challenge if the response is unsatisfactory.
- An arterial blood gas analysis will be useful in determining the net pathophysiological effect of the patient's shock. Metabolic acidosis signified by low pH, high negative base excess and elevated serum lactate is found proportionate to the severity and duration of the shock state. Serial assays are useful in assessing response to treatment.

Table 8.10 Advantages and disadvantages of direct arterial blood pressure measurement

Advantages
- Accuracy (particularly at extremes of high and low pressure)
- Continuous measurement gives immediate warning of important changes in blood pressure
- Shape of arterial waveform gives information relating to myocardial contractility and other haemodynamic variables
- Facility for frequent arterial blood sampling

Disadvantages
- Requires expertise for insertion and subsequent care
- Potentially inaccurate if apparatus is not set up correctly
- Haematoma at puncture site
- Infection at puncture site/bacteraemia/septicaemia
- Disconnection haemorrhage
- Embolization
- Arterial thrombosis

- Call for urgent senior help if the patient is not responding. Even if the patient has a satisfactory response to the fluid challenge, help will often still be required for definitive treatment.
- Increasingly, transthoracic echocardiography (TTE) is being used to diagnose a number of problems including hypovolaemia (reduced ventricular filling) and left ventricular dysfunction (see below).
- Acute haemorrhage, which may be overt or covert, must be controlled and this may require the urgent transfer of the patient to the operating theatre. The resuscitation fluid in these circumstances is blood; however, haemostasis has a higher priority than restoration of a normal blood pressure. Rapid, high volume fluid resuscitation will exacerbate bleeding and is associated with a worse prognosis.
- Hypotensive resuscitation requires the judgement of an experienced clinician.

Investigations:

- FBC, U + Es, blood glucose, CRP, coagulation screen, blood cultures (if indicated);
- blood grouping and cross-match in case of need for transfusion;

- 12-lead ECG to identify any arrhythmia or ischaemia;
- CXR to identify haemothorax, pneumothorax, heart failure, infection;
- arterial blood gas analysis to assess oxygenation, ventilation, acid base status;
- ultrasound assessment of abdomen and/or chest to identify free fluid;
- send samples of faeces for microbiological assessment.

In patients with suspected cardiac failure, early consideration should be given to invasive monitoring, for example CVP. Early use of direct arterial pressure measurement is also valuable (Table 8.10). It is now possible to use an arterial line to monitor cardiac output using a technique known as pulse contour analysis (see Chapter 2).

Sepsis and septic shock

The pathophysiology of hypotension due to sepsis is entirely different to hypovolaemic or cardiogenic shock. Any major insult to the body, such as infection, major trauma, burns, acute pancreatitis, initiates a hypermetabolic, inflammatory state termed the 'systemic inflammatory response syndrome' (SIRS). The diagnosis of SIRS is based on finding two or more of the following:

- temperature $>38\,°C$ or $<36\,°C$;
- heart rate >90 beats/min;
- respiratory rate >20 breaths/min or $PaCO_2 < 4.2\,kPa$;
- WBC count $> 12\,000/mm^3$, $< 4000/mm^3$, or >10% immature (band) forms.

Sepsis is a condition in which SIRS is due to documented or suspected infection. When the infection overwhelms the patient's immune system there is systemic spread via the blood stream (septicaemia). This triggers an inflammatory cascade, the production of inflammatory mediators that cause intense vasodilatation, capillary leak and maldistribution of blood flow at the microcirculatory level. The reflex response is an increase in sympathetic discharge causing tachycardia, increase in stroke volume and cardiac output. Despite this response there may still be hypotension (SBP < 90 mm/Hg) and evidence of hypoperfusion (lactic acidosis > 2 mmol/L, oliguria, < 0.5 mL/kg/h), this defines severe sepsis. **Septic shock is a subset of severe sepsis where there is persistent arterial hypotension (SBP**

< 90 mmHg) **and perfusion abnormalities despite adequate fluid resuscitation.** Failure to recognize and treat septic shock will result in progression to 'multiple organ dysfunction syndrome' (MODS) – the presence of altered organ function such that normal homeostasis cannot be maintained without intervention such as mechanical ventilation or renal replacement therapy. The signs of septic shock are typically:

- pyrexia;
- tachypnoea;
- warm, flushed peripheries with normal capillary refill time (CRT);
- tachycardia;
- a bounding pulse with a wide pulse pressure;
- oliguria.

Start treatment:

This is based on the Surviving Sepsis Campaign Resuscitation (6 h) bundle:

- give high-flow oxygen;
- ensure large-bore IV access;
- obtain blood cultures prior to giving antibiotics;
- give IV broad-spectrum antibiotics:
  ○ within 3 hours of admission to the emergency department;
  ○ within 1 hour for an inpatient.

Early antibiotic therapy is strongly associated with improved survival and is even more important than fluid resuscitation.

- Take an arterial blood sample and measure serum lactate to assess the severity of septic shock:
  ○ a lactate level > 2 mmol/L is indicative of severe sepsis;
- Treat hypotension/raised lactate (>2 mmol/L) with fluids:
  ○ initial fluid bolus of 20 ml/kg crystalloid or equivalent volume of colloid.

Loss of fluid through leaky capillaries may lead to excessively high volumes of acute resuscitation fluids – sometimes over 5 L over a period of several hours. Continual fluid infusion will inevitably lead to pulmonary interstitial and alveolar oedema, respiratory distress and hypoxaemia – acute respiratory distress syndrome (ARDS).

- Start vasopressors if hypotension doesn't respond to fluid resuscitation, maintain MAP > 65 mmHg:

  ○ the vasodilated circulation often responds well to an intravenous infusion of a vasopressor agent such as noradrenaline.
- Achieve and maintain:
  ○ CVP > 8 mmHg;
  ○ central venous oxygen saturation ($ScvO_2$) > 70%.

Patients who do not show an improvement in tissue perfusion with fluid resuscitation (those with septic shock) will need to be managed in a critical care unit where a vasopressor can be used and invasive haemodynamic monitoring can be instituted.

Cardiogenic shock

Patients with cardiogenic shock due to acute heart failure associated with an acute coronary syndrome (ACS) are managed differently, so it is essential to make the correct diagnosis. This will often come from the clinical context of the patient's illness and any typical physical signs present. Management of the hypotension is covered below and management of the ACS is covered in the relevant section below.

Most patients with cardiogenic shock will present with left ventricular failure that can be described as:

- 'Forward failure' – a decrease in stroke volume and cardiac output. Symptoms and signs include:
  ○ pallor, peripheral cyanosis, cold extremities, delayed capillary refill, oliguria, altered conscious level, gallop rhythm.
- 'Backward failure' – acute dilatation of the left side of the heart and accumulation of blood in the pulmonary circulation that promotes the development of acute pulmonary oedema. Symptoms and signs include:
  ○ dyspnoea, wheeze, cough with pink frothy sputum, cyanosis, basal crackles in the lungs, displaced apex beat.

Frequently, both types of failure coexist.

- In some patients with acute inferior myocardial infarction when the predominant problem may be failure of the right rather than the left ventricle. Symptoms and signs include:
  ○ peripheral oedema, jugular vein distension, hepatomegaly (tender), ascites, pleural effusion.

Start treatment:

- This will consist initially of treatment of pulmonary oedema as described above.

- Patients with poor cardiac output are not usually hypovolaemic and do not respond favourably to a fluid challenge as this compounds the problem of excessive filling pressure.
- Inotropic support with dobutamine may be required to improve contractility of the left ventricle and this will need the patient to be transferred to a critical or coronary care unit for invasive monitoring.
- Where monitoring can be used to confirm adequate or excessive left ventricular filling pressures, diuretic and vasodilator therapy can be used to improve cardiac output.
- Patients with predominant right heart failure are the exception to the withhold fluids rule – poor performance of the right ventricle leads to underfilling of the left ventricle and a fluid challenge may be beneficial.

Investigations:

- CXR may show cardiomegaly, pulmonary congestion, Kerley B lines, loss of costophrenic angles.
- 12-lead ECG may show evidence of ischaemia or an arrhythmia (see below).
- Echocardiography will reveal left and right ventricular dysfunction (ischaemia, cardiomyopathy), valvular disease.
- Blood tests as above plus markers of myocardial infarction (cardiac troponins).

Low urine output

The obligatory minimum daily urine output consistent with maintaining normal homeostasis is approximately 500 mL. If urine output falls below this level, or if the kidneys are incapable of producing urine of appropriate concentration for the volume produced, renal failure results. Oliguria is usually defined as $< 0.5\,mL/kg/h$. Anuria is the complete absence of urine production; this cannot be diagnosed with certainty unless the patient is catheterized. However, it is essential to recognize that the commonest cause of anuria in an already catheterized patient is a blocked catheter! Palpation over the lower abdomen of an anuric, catheterized patient may confirm the diagnosis. Regardless, the urinary catheter of all such patients should be either flushed or replaced.

Table 8.11 Aetiology of acute kidney injury

Pre-renal
- Dehydration, e.g. vomiting, diarrhoea
- Haemorrhage
- Cardiogenic shock
- 'Third-space losses', e.g. trauma, major surgery, bowel obstruction
- Sepsis
- Burns

Renal
- Acute tubular necrosis (usually secondary to severe pre-renal failure)
- Sepsis
- Severe obstructive jaundice
- Blood transfusion reaction
- Myoglobinaemia secondary to ischaemic muscle damage and rhabdomyolysis
- Acute glomerular disorders
- Infection, e.g. acute pyelonephritis
- Vasculitis

Post-Renal
- Bilateral obstruction to renal outflow (e.g. tumour)

For patients on general wards, the most important causes of oliguria are:

- Hypovolaemia usually as a result of:
  - inadequate fluid intake to meet needs;
  - losses from drains, gastrointestinal tract (vomiting, diarrhoea, fistulae);
  - third space losses after major surgery;
  - haemorrhage;
  - sepsis.
- Stress response to surgery (see Chapter 7).

Failure to recognize and treat hypovolaemia will lead to the development of pre-renal acute kidney injury (AKI). If diagnosed and treated promptly, particularly with sufficient volume resuscitation, pre-renal AKI often resolves and urine output increases. The aetiology of AKI can also be renal or post-renal. The causes are summarized in Table 8.11.

Similarly post-renal AKI is potentially reversible if recognized early enough and the obstruction relieved, which may be as simple as catheterizing the patient.

Patients suffering from an inadequate fluid intake will have signs and symptoms of dehydration, the severity of which will depend on the fluid deficit:

- <10% loss body weight:
  - thirst, dry mouth;
  - tachycardia;
  - empty peripheral and central veins (low CVP);
  - reduced skin turgour;
- >10% loss body weight:
  - as above plus increased respiratory rate, hypotension, anuria, delirium, coma.

A review of the patient's fluid balance charts will often reveal trends of increasing pulse rate, decreasing urine output, falling blood pressure and increasing respiratory rate.

Start treatment:

When asked to see a patient on the ward who is oliguric, the initial approach must be directed at identifying and treating any airway, breathing and circulation problems.

- *Hypoxaemia:* Immediate treatment with oxygen as described above.
- *Hypotension:* Identify the likely cause and treat as described above. In most cases this will require fluid resuscitation. There will be a delay after appropriate resuscitation has been provided before urine production increases – resist the temptation to give a dose of a diuretic, for example furosemide, which does not have a useful place in the treatment of pre-renal failure.
- *Exclude a post-renal cause urgently:* This is usually done by excluding urinary retention clinically, ensuring that a urinary catheter, if present, is not blocked.
- *Stop all nephrotoxic drugs:* These include NSAIDs, aminoglycosides, and angiotensin converting enzyme (ACE) inhibitors. Paracetamol is safe in the acute setting.

Any condition that precipitated acute pre-renal failure must be treated, for example sepsis secondary to perforated abdominal viscus requires urgent surgical referral for a laparotomy.

Investigations:

- FBC will usually show an increased haematocrit due to dehydration and raised white cell count if infection is present;
- plasma U + Es and creatinine; will normally show an increase in plasma sodium and urea but little increase in creatinine;
- urine sodium is reduced (Table 8.12);
- plasma and urine osmolalities will show a high urinary to plasma osmolality, often >1.5:1;
- ultrasound of the kidneys and ureters to exclude obstruction to urine flow.

As stated above, failure to recognize and treat these problems will lead to AKI and the development of acute tubular necrosis (ATN). Diagnosis is predominantly based on the history and investigations:

- taking a blood sample for U + Es and creatinine;
- estimated GFR (eGFR);
- measured creatinine clearance;
- urinalysis.

Raised serum urea and creatinine are synonymous with renal failure. However, it is important to be wary of several pitfalls:

- Normal values may not be normal for specific patient groups. A frail, elderly patient's serum creatinine concentration may be within normal limits, but may in fact reflect abnormal renal function.

Table 8.12 Differentiation of pre-renal from intrinsic renal failure

Index	Pre-renal	Intrinsic renal
Urine concentration	High	Dilute
Specific gravity	≥1020	<1010
Osmolarity (mosmol/L)	>550	<350
Urine [Na] (mmol/L)	<20	>40
Urine/plasma osmolar ratio	≥2:1	1.1:1
Urine/plasma [urea]	≥20:1	<10:1
Urine/plasma [creatinine]	≥40:1	<10:1
Plasma [urea] (mmol/L)/ [creatinine] (μmol/L) ratio	>0.1	<0.1

- A single U + E estimation is a snapshot of renal function and is only reliable when renal function is stable. A patient who has become acutely oliguric may have normal values.
- Many laboratories provide an estimate of GFR (eGFR). This is estimated using an algorithm based often only on the patient's age, sex and weight. It is not valid in an acute situation where the serum creatinine is in the process of either rising or falling.
- Renal function has to be severely impaired for the numbers to change. Serum creatinine only starts to rise significantly above the normal range when GFR falls below about 30 mL/min (normal 125 mL/min). A modestly elevated creatinine indicates quite severe loss of global renal function.
- There could be other reasons for a rising urea; in dehydrated patients a urea concentration relatively higher than the creatinine may indicate dehydration without AKI. In upper GI bleeding high levels of protein breakdown leads to increased urea production with raised serum concentrations. All of these conditions also predispose to AKI.

Urinalysis will show dilute urine, with a low osmolality (urine:plasma ratio, 1.1:1) (Table 8.12). Urine microscopy may show the presence of casts (indicative of acute tubular necrosis and glomerulonephritis) and micro-organisms (urinary sepsis is a common cause of AKI). However, urinalysis is not useful for diagnosing whether or not pre-renal failure is the cause (Table 8.12).

A patient with raised serum urea and creatinine who is developing or has established acute renal failure should be transferred to a critical care unit to allow central venous pressure, direct arterial pressure and cardiac output monitoring. These will guide fluid therapy more reliably. If required the patient can be commenced on renal replacement therapy (RRT) with continuous veno-venous haemo-filtration, an extracorporeal renal support therapy similar in some ways to the more familiar intermittent haemodialysis.

If pre-renal and post-renal causes are excluded, there is likely to be a significant intrinsic renal problem. These patients will require urgent specialist nephrologist help with investigation and management.

Chest pain

As already described, many acute problems present with chest pain as a feature. This section will concentrate on chest pain that is a result of the patient suffering an acute coronary syndrome (ACS); unstable angina, non-ST-segment-elevation myocardial infarction (NSTEMI) and ST-segment-elevation myocardial infarction (STEMI). The pain is indicative of myocardial ischaemia or infarction, caused by the formation of thrombus that partially or completely occludes a coronary artery. The symptoms and signs consistent with acute myocardial ischaemia or infarction (AMI) include:

- central chest pain, often described as dull or constricting;
- the pain often radiates to the neck, jaw, the left or both arms, or epigastrium;
- nausea and vomiting;
- pallor;
- sweating;
- tachycardia;
- dyspnoea;
- heart failure.

Although the pain described above is typical, it is not necessarily ubiquitous. The elderly, diabetics and postoperative patients may have no chest pain.

Unstable angina

The diagnosis depends on finding one or more of:

- angina on exertion, provoked by progressively less activity;
- angina occurring without provocation;
- prolonged angina suggesting myocardial infarction, but no ECG or laboratory evidence of myocardial infarction.

The 12-lead ECG may be:

- normal;
- show ST segment depression;
- show T wave inversion.

There is no elevation of serum cardiac troponins or cardiac enzymes.

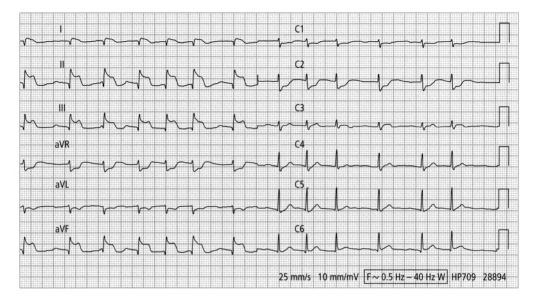

Figure 8.5 Twelve-lead ECG showing an STEMI; inferior myocardial infarction with ST elevation in leads II, III and aVF.

Non-ST-segment-elevation myocardial infarction (NSTEMI)

The diagnosis depends on finding:

- chest pain as described above, usually lasting for more than 20 min;
- non-specific ECG changes – ST segment depression or T wave inversion on the 12-lead ECG;
- raised plasma concentrations of cardiac troponins.

ST-segment-elevation myocardial infarction (STEMI) (Fig. 8.5)

The diagnosis depends on finding:

- chest pain as described above, usually lasting for more than 20 min;
- ST segment elevation or new left bundle branch block (LBBB) on a 12-lead ECG;
- raised plasma concentrations of cardiac troponins.

Although the release of cardiac troponins is evidence of myocardial infarction, alone it is not diagnostic, as they can be released in many of the other acute conditions described so far including pulmonary embolism, heart failure, renal failure and sepsis.

Start treatment

All patients suffering an ACS should immediately be given:

- aspirin, 300 mg orally, crushed or chewed;
- nitrates, usually sublingual GTN, unless hypotensive;
- oxygen, high flow initially, titrated to a SpO_2 94–98% once it can be monitored;
- analgesia, usually IV diamorphine, titrated to relieve pain.

Patients suffering from unstable angina or NSTEMI will need urgent treatment to prevent the spread of coronary thrombus:

- low molecular weight heparin or fondaparinux, subcutaneously, in a therapeutic dose;
- clopidogrel, if no contraindication;
- consider a glycoprotein IIb/IIIa inhibitor if early PCI is planned (see below).

If not contraindicated, a beta-blocker should be given to reduce myocardial oxygen demand and if there is evidence of heart failure, early introduction of an ACE inhibitor and a statin.

All patients should be cared for in an area with continuous ECG monitoring and immediate availability of a defibrillator. Patients should be referred urgently for consideration of coronary angiography to determine the need for coronary revascularization.

Patients who have sustained a STEMI will require urgent referral for coronary reperfusion therapy, either by primary percutaneous coronary intervention (PCI) or fibrinolytic therapy. Typical indications for immediate reperfusion therapy are:

- presentation within 12 hours of onset of chest pain suggesting AMI and;
- ST segment elevation >0.2 mV in 2 adjacent chest leads or >0.1 mV in two adjacent limb leads, or;
- dominant R waves and ST depression in leads V1-V3 or;
- new or presumed new-onset LBBB.

Cardiac arrhythmias

Any arrhythmia can cause acute cardiovascular compromise as the effectiveness of the heart as a pump is reduced therefore reducing cardiac output. Arrhythmias can arise for a number of reasons, the most common precipitants being:

- structural heart disease – for example, cardio-myopathy, left ventricular hypertrophy, valve disease;
- myocardial ischaemia;
- electrolyte abnormality, particularly potassium and magnesium;
- hypovolaemia;
- sepsis;
- side effects of other drugs.

Often it is a combination of factors, for example electrolyte disturbance in the presence of long-standing left-ventricular hypertrophy.

Following the initial assessment of the patient, assuming the presence of a cardiac output, the next steps are as follows:

- Give high flow oxygen if not already in place.
- Make sure full resuscitation equipment is immediately to hand.
- Establish adequate IV access and take bloods.
- Establish continuous ECG monitoring – this is probably best done through defibrillator pads.
- Identify the exact nature of the arrhythmia.
- Determine the degree of cardiovascular compromise and the urgency of treatment.
- Administer the appropriate treatment for the arrhythmia.

- Correct any predisposing factors such as electrolytes, hypoxia, hypovolaemia.
- Following treatment obtain a 12-lead ECG.
- Arrange appropriate ongoing management and monitoring, for example in a coronary care unit or ITU.

Arrhythmias can cause a variable amount of compromise depending on the exact nature of the rhythm, the heart rate, and the presence of any pre-existing cardiac disease. The urgency of the situation, and hence the appropriate management will be dictated by the patient's clinical condition. Adverse features indicating an unstable patient who is at risk of deterioration and who needs urgent treatment and senior help are as follows:

- Extreme heart rates – rates >150/min or <40/min are generally poorly tolerated.
- Shock – systolic BP <90 mmHg, poor peripheral perfusion.
- Syncope – signifying impaired cerebral perfusion.
- Heart failure – the presence of pulmonary oedema.
- Myocardial ischaemia – chest pain or ECG changes suggesting ischaemia.

More specific management directed at restoring a normal heart rate and/or rhythm can be started once the underlying rhythm abnormality and the urgency are known. The following are based on the Resuscitation Council (UK) 2011 guidelines.

Tachycardias

These can be divided based on the duration of the QRS complex on the ECG into:

- narrow complex tachycardias (QRS < 0.12 s) – supra-ventricular in origin.
- broad complex tachycardias (QRS > 0.12 s) – these can be ventricular in origin or supra-ventricular tachycardia with an abnormal conduction pathway.

If in doubt as to the exact cause of a broad complex tachycardia treat it as ventricular tachycardia.

Patients **with any adverse features** will need synchronized cardioversion under sedation or general anaesthesia and an anaesthetist should be called for this. Up to three shocks of increasing energy may be delivered. The starting energy level needed for cardioversion depends upon the type of arrhythmia:

- Broad complex or atrial fibrillation – 120–150 J biphasic and increase in increments.
- Regular narrow complex and atrial flutter – 70–120 J biphasic.

If the arrhythmia is not terminated after three shocks, give 300 mg Amiodarone IV over 10–20 min followed by another single shock.

If the patient **does not have any adverse features** there are other treatment options:

- Narrow complex, regular – likely to be a supraventricular tachycardia (SVT), try vagal manoeuvres (carotid sinus massage, valsalva manoeuvre). If these fail give up to three adenosine boluses (6 mg, 12 mg, 12 mg). If sinus rhythm is not restored then more expert help will be needed.
- Narrow complex, irregular – likely to be atrial fibrillation; give atenolol 5 mg IV.
- Broad complex, regular – probable ventricular tachycardia (VT), give amiodarone 300 mg IV over 20–60 min, followed by 900 mg over 24 hours (via a central line).
- Broad complex, irregular – obtain expert help as it will probably be difficult to determine the underlying rhythm.

Bradycardia

If there are any adverse features present:

- Give atropine 500 μg IV immediately.
- This can be repeated until a satisfactory heart rate and blood pressure are achieved, or up to a maximum dose of 3 mg.
- If there is an inadequate response to atropine then an adrenaline infusion or transcutaneous pacing can be started.
- Adrenaline- or transcutaneous pacing-dependent patients will subsequently require transvenous pacing and specialist cardiology help should be obtained urgently.

If there are no adverse features present:

- Assess the risk of deterioration to asystole – high risk of this is associated with:
  ○ recent asystole;
  ○ Mobitz type 2 AV block;
  ○ complete heart block with broad QRS complex;
  ○ ventricular pause >3 s.
- If a high risk is present, treat as above and obtain expert help.
- If there are no high-risk features, the patient can be monitored.

Cardiac arrest

Unfortunately, significant numbers of patients in hospital will have a cardiac arrest either as a result of primary cardiac disease or as the end point of unrecognized physiological deterioration. All healthcare professionals need to be competent to deal with a patient who has had a cardiac arrest, either as a first responder or as a member of the cardiac arrest team. The details below are based on the guidelines produced by the Resuscitation Council (UK).

Members of the team responding to a cardiac arrest call should ideally meet at the beginning of their period of duty and carry out a number of tasks, including:

- introductions by name;
- identification of skills and experience;
- allocate team leader responsibility;
- allocate roles, for example airway management, defibrillation;
- identify any deficiencies and how they can be managed – for example, if nobody is able to perform tracheal intubation;
- ensure that everyone is aware of the need for personal safety – for example, use of gloves and need for ANTT techniques;
- the need to ensure audit is performed;
- arrangements for debriefing.

Actions on attending a cardiac arrest

On most occasions in hospital, resuscitation will have been started by other healthcare professionals before the team arrives. A standardized approach to management of cardiac arrest is used, dependent on the initial rhythm, either shockable (VF/VT) or non-shockable (pulseless electrical activity (PEA) or asystole). This is summarized in Fig. 8.6.

- Confirm cardiac arrest, check for breathing and a central pulse simultaneously (Fig. 8.7).
- Ensure good-quality CPR (compression-ventilation ratio 30:2) (Fig. 8.8):
  ○ Chest compressions; heel of hands in middle of lower half of sternum, depth 5–6 cm, rate 100–120/min, ensure complete release between compressions. Use a CPR feedback or prompt device if available.
  ○ Ventilation – use a bag-mask alone or with a supraglottic airway device. If the skills are

available, perform tracheal intubation. Ventilate at 10 breaths/min.

○ Attach self-adhesive defibrillator pads while chest compressions are ongoing (Fig. 8.9).

• Once the airway is secure, attempt uninterrupted compressions and ventilations.

• Plan actions for team members to minimize hands-off time if defibrillation is required.

• Stop CPR and check rhythm on monitor, immediately resume CPR. Take less than 10 s.

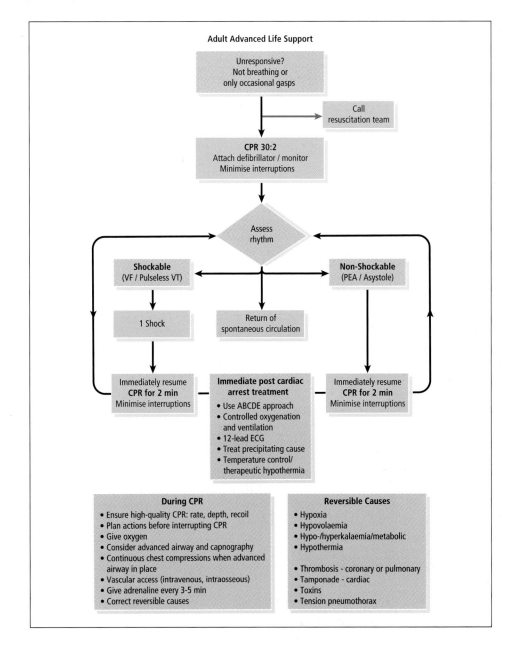

Figure 8.6 Adult Advanced Life Support (ALS) algorithm. Courtesy of the Resuscitation Council (UK).

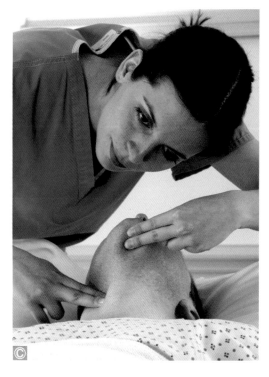

Figure 8.7 Simultaneous check of breathing and pulse to confirm cardiac arrest. Picture courtesy of Dr Mike Scott and Resuscitation Council (UK).

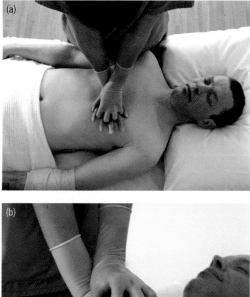

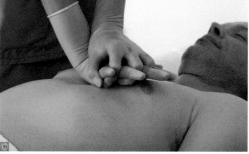

Figure 8.8 (a, b) Chest compressions during CPR. Note hand position in the middle of the lower half of the sternum. Courtesy of Dr Mike Scott and Resuscitation Council UK.

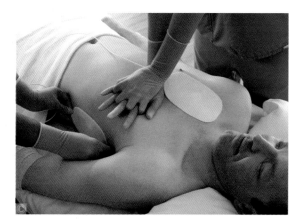

Figure 8.9 Self-adhesive pads being applied with on-going chest compressions. Courtesy of Dr Mike Scott and Resuscitation Council (UK).

If VF or VT:

1 Designated person selects correct energy on the defibrillator; 150–200 J biphasic for first shock, 150–360 J for subsequent shocks, and charges defibrillator.
2 During charging, warn all team members to stand clear, **except the person doing chest compressions,** and remove any device delivering oxygen.
3 Once the defibrillator is charged, warn person doing chest compressions to stand clear. **When clear deliver shock**.
4 Without checking rhythm or pulse immediately recommence CPR.
5 Continue CPR for 2 min, team leader prepares for actions during next pause.

- After 2 min, check the monitor:
  ○ if a rhythm compatible with a cardiac output is seen, check for signs of a circulation, such as pulse or increase in $ETCO_2$;
  ○ if VF persists, repeat steps 1 to 5.
- After 2 min, check the monitor:
  ○ if a rhythm compatible with a cardiac output is seen, check for signs of a circulation;
  ○ if VF persists, repeat steps 1 to 4;
  ○ give 1 mg adrenaline IV and 300 mg amiodarone IV while performing CPR.
- Repeat the 2 min sequence of CPR-rhythm check-defibrillation while VF persists.
- Give further doses of 1 mg adrenaline every alternate shock, approximately every 3–5 min.
- In shock-refractory VF, identify and treat any reversible causes that may be contributing, such as hyperkalaemia.
- If the patient has a return of spontaneous circulation (ROSC), organize post-resuscitation care. This will require transfer of the patient to a critical care area.
- If the rhythm changes to asystole or electrical activity without a perfusing rhythm, switch to the non-shockable side of the algorithm (see below).

If PEA or asystole:

- Give adrenaline 1 mg IV.
- During 2 min CPR, secure the airway if not already done.
- After 2 min check rhythm, if organized electrical activity is seen, check for signs of a circulation:
  ○ if there is ROSC, organize post-resuscitation care;
  ○ if there is no ROSC, continue CPR for 2 min, give further doses of adrenaline every 3–5 min;

○ recheck the rhythm check every 2 min;
○ if there is a change to VF/VT at the rhythm check, change to the shockable side of the algorithm.
- While CPR is ongoing, identify and treat any reversible causes (4Hs and 4Ts):
  ○ hypoxia;
  ○ hypovolaemia;
  ○ hypo-/hyperkalaemia/metabolic disturbances;
  ○ hypothermia;
  ○ thrombosis – coronary or pulmonary;
  ○ tamponade – cardiac;
  ○ toxins – for example, drug overdose;
  ○ tension pneumothorax.

If resuscitation is unsuccessful, the team leader should lead a discussion on stopping the attempt with all team members. This will require judgement based upon the patient's premorbid status, current rhythm, response so far to the resuscitation, and likelihood of ROSC if continuing the attempt. Confirmation of death occurs approximately 5 min after stopping CPR by confirming that there is no evidence of a central pulse and no heart sounds on auscultation.

At the end of every cardiac arrest, it is the team leader's responsibility that appropriate audit data is collected and recorded.

KEY POINTS

- Ensure good-quality CPR is performed at all times. Change the person performing CPR regularly to prevent fatigue.
- Minimize delays between stopping compressions and delivering the shock – ideally less than 5 s.
- Resume chest compressions after shock delivery. Even if a perfusing rhythm has been restored, a pulse may not be palpable.
- If an organized rhythm is seen during the 2 min period of CPR, do not stop chest compressions unless the patient shows signs of life.
- In shock refractory VF, check the position and contact of the pads.
- If there is doubt whether the rhythm is fine VF or asystole, do not attempt defibrillation – continue CPR. This may improve the amplitude of VF and increase the chance of successful defibrillation

Reduced conscious level

This may be due to a number of causes. The treatment priorities remain:

- establishing and maintaining a patent airway;
- ensuring adequate oxygenation and ventilation;
- supporting or restoring an adequate circulation;
- assessing the GCS.

Then proceed to determine the cause of the depressed consciousness. Some of the more common causes, and their management, are outlined below.

Hypoglycaemia

This is most likely in patients with diabetes receiving oral hypoglycaemic agents or insulin treatment. It can occur in the perioperative period if there is inadequate carbohydrate intake or absorption but normal doses of medication are continued, and in those developing sepsis. Patients with poorly controlled diabetes may become symptomatic at what would otherwise be considered normal blood glucose concentrations. Other groups of patients at risk are those with hepatic failure, who have impaired hepatic gluconeogenesis during starvation, and those who have had a gastrectomy. The brain is dependent on a constant supply of glucose for energy and so untreated hypoglycaemia has the potential to cause irreversible brain damage.

The presenting features depend on blood sugar concentration and are due to autonomic stimulation and inadequate glucose delivery to the brain:

- autonomic – sweating, tachycardia, tremor, hunger:
  - patients taking beta-blockers may not have any of the autonomic signs or symptoms of hypoglycaemia;
- inadequate cerebral glucose delivery – delirium, reduced GCS, seizures.

Details within the patient's medical history may raise suspicion of the diagnosis, and a conscious patient may describe the classical symptoms listed above. The diagnosis is confirmed by checking a capillary blood glucose concentration. All patients with a decreased GCS should have a capillary blood glucose checked as part of their initial assessment.

Start treatment

The key aims are to increase the blood glucose concentration back to normal levels, and prevent further hypoglycaemic episodes.

If the patient has a patent airway, is breathing and conscious:

- give oral glucose gel, for example hypostop – glucose is rapidly absorbed across the buccal membranes;
- obtain IV access;
- the oral glucose alone may not be enough, and a bolus of 250–500 mL 10% dextrose IV may be needed.

If the patient is unconscious:

- ensure a patent airway and adequate ventilation;
- obtain IV access and give 25–50 g of dextrose as an IV dextrose solution:
  - 50% dextrose is often stored on resuscitation trolleys, but causes phlebitis;
  - 10% dextrose is preferable as this causes less irritation;
- a rapid recovery is often seen.

Calculating the dose of dextrose in grams from percentage:

$$\text{concentration } (\%) \times 10 \times \text{volume (L)} = \text{dose (g)}$$

e.g. 500 mL of 10% solution

$$10\% \times 10 \times 0.5\,\text{L} = 50\,\text{g}$$

Investigations:

- 12-lead ECG to check for any myocardial ischaemia or arrhythmia;
- blood tests, including FBC, U + Es, blood sugar and blood cultures.

Once the blood glucose concentration has been restored to normal the symptoms should have resolved. If there is ongoing neurological impairment an alternative explanation should be sought. Further episodes can be prevented by:

- the patient taking an oral diet:
  - immediate and slow-release carbohydrate, for example sugary drink and toast;
  - consider altering dose of regular diabetes medication;
- the patient not taking oral diet or not absorbing enteral nutrition:

- o intravenous insulin and dextrose infusions either as a sliding scale or an 'Alberti regime' according to local guidelines;
- o stop normal diabetes medication until normal oral diet has been resumed;
- all patients must have frequent monitoring of capillary blood glucose until the 'at risk' period is over.

Opioid narcosis

Opioids form a key part of the management of moderate and severe acute post-operative pain. A variety of different opioids are in common use and they can be administered via a number of different routes – for example, oral, IV, intrathecal or epidural. There is also a wide inter-individual variability in the metabolism and elimination of opioids, which leads to the potential for overdose. The elderly, patients with obstructive sleep apnoea and patients with altered renal function are particularly at risk. Specific features of opioid overdose include:

- History – receiving opioids, elderly, abnormal renal function.
- Hypoventilation – particularly reduced respiratory rate.
- Pupils – 'pin-point' in appearance.

Start treatment:

- ensure an adequate airway, breathing and circulation;
- establish IV access if not already in place;
- give naloxone, in 100–200 µg boluses IV until an adequate conscious level and respiratory rate are restored.

Naloxone also reverses the analgesic effects of the opioids. The aim is that with careful titration the harmful side-effects can be reversed without antagonizing all the analgesia.

The effects of naloxone are relatively short lived (approximately 20 min). Therefore, if long-acting opioids have been given, such as morphine, or opioids have been given intrathecally, repeat naloxone doses or an infusion may be needed, as well as adequate monitoring, which may necessitate admission to a critical care unit.

Stroke/intracranial haemorrhage

A stroke may occur for a number of different reasons including, but not limited to:

- atrial fibrillation – emboli from atrial thrombus;
- severe hypotension – due to haemorrhage or sepsis;
- a period of hypoxaemia – due to respiratory depression from opioids;
- intracranial haemorrhage – due to anticoagulation with heparin;
- related to surgery – emboli following carotid endarterectomy.

The clinical features and appropriate management depend upon the extent and the location of the cerebral damage:

- if there is infarction of a large volume of cerebral tissue, or a large intracranial haematoma, the patient's GCS will be reduced, and the patient may not be able to maintain a patent airway;
- small areas of infarct may give rise to only localized motor or sensory deficits with a preserved GCS.

Start treatment:

- ensure an adequate airway, breathing and circulation;
- give supplemental oxygen; if $SpO_2 < 94\%$, aim for 94–98%.

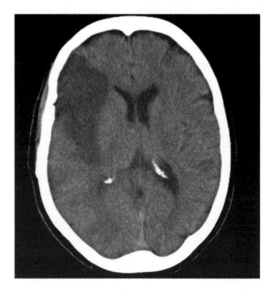

Figure 8.10 CT brain showing large low density area in the right fronto-parietal region, consistent with an ischaemic stroke.

Following the initial assessment and stabilization the priorities are:

- An urgent CT scan of the head to confirm the diagnosis (Fig. 8.10). This may necessitate intubation and ventilation to be performed safely:
  - some centres are performing thrombolysis for ischaemic strokes confirmed by CT scan within 3 hours of onset of symptoms – in these cases time is of the essence;
  - thrombolysis may be contraindicated in the postoperative period.
- If intracranial haemorrhage is excluded by CT scan, 300 mg aspirin should be given as soon as possible.
- Control blood glucose concentrations. Use a glucose and insulin infusion if needed; a target of 4–11 mmol/L is recommended.
- Blood pressure control is only indicated if there are other problems, such as intracerebral haemorrhage or myocardial infarction, or if thrombolysis is planned.
- Conscious patients should have a swallowing assessment; nasogastric feeding should be started within 24 hours in patients unable to swallow safely.
- Involve the acute stroke team early.

If the CT scan shows an intracranial haemorrhage the patient will need to be discussed with the local neurosurgical unit to determine if surgical management will be beneficial. If the patient is on anti-coagulant therapy there may be some difficult decisions about the relative risks and benefits of continuing or stopping treatment. Further management will depend on the neurosurgical opinion.

Status epilepticus

Status epilepticus is defined as seizures lasting more than 30 min, or frequent seizures over 30 min without a return to consciousness. The aim of treatment is to terminate seizures as quickly as possible because of the high mortality associated with them, and this usually requires intravenous antiepileptic drugs or, if refractory, general anaesthesia. Early expert help is therefore essential.

The common causes of status epilepticus include:

- unstable, poorly controlled epilepsy;
- acute brain injury: stroke, tumour, subarachnoid haemorrhage, trauma, hypoxia;
- previous brain injury: trauma, neurosurgery, arteriovenous malformations;
- CNS infection: encephalitis, meningitis, abscess;
- metabolic abnormalities: hypoglycaemia, hyponatraemia, hypocalcaemia, uraemia;
- sub-therapeutic antiepileptic drug levels in known epileptics;
- withdrawal syndromes: alcohol, barbiturates or benzodiazepines;
- eclampsia of pregnancy;
- febrile convulsions may precipitate status epilepticus in young children (3 months to 3 years of age).

Start treatment:

- Clear and maintain an airway. This may be difficult. A nasopharyngeal airway is often very useful due to clenching of the jaw during the fit.
- Give high-flow oxygen via a facemask with reservoir.
- Establish IV access and take blood for immediate glucose analysis.
- Correct hypotension with IV fluids.
- Start antiepileptic therapy IV:
  - first-line therapy, IV lorazepam up to 4.0 mg;
  - if IV access not possible, diazepam 10 mg PR (this may already have been given by paramedics prehospital).

If seizures continue:

- IV phenytoin 15 mg/kg at a rate of ≤50 mg/min.
  - ECG monitoring is essential as risk of bradycardia and heart block.
- IV sodium valproate 10 mg/kg at a rate of ≤100 mg/min (followed by 1.6 g over 24 hours).

Refractory status epilepticus:

- Induce and maintain general anaesthesia with tracheal intubation. This will require expert help.

Investigations:

- Plasma glucose, U&Es, calcium, magnesium, FBC, therapeutic drug levels, toxicology screen, arterial blood gases.
- Septic screen, including lumbar puncture if CNS infection suspected.
- CT scan. The possibility of intracranial pathology is high if this is the first presentation of epilepsy.
- EEG.

As soon as seizures are controlled, refer the patient to a neurologist.

Reduced level of consciousness secondary to hypoxaemia or hypovolaemia

The brain requires a constant supply of oxygen for its normal function. Both hypoxaemia and hypovolaemia will compromise cerebral oxygen delivery. Both of these abnormalities should have been detected and treated during the initial ABCDE assessment of the patient, and some signs of increasing cerebral function may be seen within minutes of appropriate management.

It must be remembered that hypoxaemia or hypovolaemia may themselves be due to another problem; for example, hypoxaemia may be due to pneumonia or pneumothorax, and hypovolaemia may be the result of intra-abdominal bleeding postoperatively. Initial measures may temporarily restore cerebral oxygenation, but definitive treatment needs to be targeted towards the underlying problem, for example intubation and mechanical ventilation, while the pneumonia resolves with antimicrobial therapy, drainage of the pneumothorax, or return to theatre to stop the bleeding.

📖 FURTHER USEFUL INFORMATION

British Thoracic Society guidelines for Management of Suspected Acute Pulmonary Embolism. *Thorax* 2003; **58**; 470–84.

National Institute for Health and Clinical Excellence. Clinical Guideline 68. *Diagnosis and initial management of acute stroke and transient ischaemic attack (TIA).* July 2008. London: NICE.

National Institute for Health and Clinical Excellence. *Clinical Guideline 94. Unstable angina and NSTEMI: the early management of unstable angina and non-ST-segment-elevation myocardial infarction.* March 2010. London: NICE.

Ramrakha P, Moore K, Sam A (eds) *Oxford handbook of acute medicine.* 3rd edn. Oxford: Oxford University Press, 2010.

The British Thoracic Society and the Scottish Intercollegiate Guideline Network. *British Guideline on the Management of Asthma: a national clinical guideline.* Revised May 2011. London and Edinburgh, 2008, revised May 2011.

The British Thoracic Society guideline for emergency oxygen use in adult patients. *Thorax* 2008; **63** (supplement VI): vi1–vi68.

The British Thoracic Society guideline for the management of community acquired pneumonia in adults: update 2009. *Thorax* 2009; **64** (supplement III); iii1–iii55.

Resuscitation Council (UK) *Adult advanced life support manual.* London: Resuscitation Council (UK), 2011.

http://bestbets.org/
[This website contains best evidence topic reviews for emergency medicine. Many of these are relevant to anaesthesia and critically ill patients.]

www.brit-thoracic.org.uk/Portals/0/Guidelines/AsthmaGuidelines/qrg101%20revised%202009.pdf
[A quick reference guide for the management of asthma in adults and children.]

www.cprguidelines.eu/2010/
[This site contains all the scientific data supporting the current guidelines for cardio-pulmonary resuscitation.]

https://www.erc.edu/
[European Resuscitation Council website.]

www.nice.org.uk/CG50
[Recognition of and response to acute illness in adults in hospital. July 2007. The NICE guidelines–you must read this if you are interested in this topic.]

www.renal.org/Clinical/GuidelinesSection/AcuteKidneyInjury.aspx
[The Renal Association website with the current guidelines for management of Acute Kidney Injury]

www.resus.org.uk
[The Resuscitation Council UK. This site contains the current UK guidelines for cardio-pulmonary resuscitation.]

www.survivingsepsis.org
[Comprehensive website run by the European Society of Intensive Care Medicine aimed at improving recognition and management of sepsis.]

www.tracheostomy.org.uk
[New organization aiming to reduce preventable deaths from mismanagement of blocked tracheostomies and laryngectomies]

All websites last accessed February 2012.

? SELF-ASSESSMENT

Short-answer questions

8.1 How would you assess a patient for signs of airway obstruction? What would be your immediate management of this problem?

8.2 A 22-year-old male on the orthopaedic ward, who is a known asthmatic, becomes increasingly breathless and wheezy one hour after an uneventful arthroscopy of his knee. He has used his salbutamol inhaler with no effect and when you arrive he is having difficulty completing sentences. What would your immediate management consist of?

8.3 You are called to a medical ward to see a patient who has suddenly deteriorated and is now unresponsive. When you arrive, a nurse is doing chest compressions. What are your immediate actions?

8.4 What symptoms and signs would suggest sepsis in a patient, 48 hours after a laparotomy? What would be your management in the first hour?

8.5 You are called about a 67-year-old woman who had an uncomplicated hip replacement 24 hours ago and has only passed 100 mL urine in the last 6 hours. What is your immediate management? What are the most likely causes?

8.6 You are called to see a 70-year-old man on the day care unit who has had lower GI endoscopy under sedation. He is known to suffer from ischaemic heart disease and he is now complaining of severe angina, feeling nauseated and slightly short of breath. On arrival he appears pale, sweaty and has a weak radial pulse. What is the most likely diagnosis? What treatment and investigations will you perform in the next 30 minutes?

True/false questions

8.1 During the initial assessment of an acutely unwell adult patient:

a a full assessment of the patient should be made before beginning any intervention/treatment;

b measuring SpO_2 helps assesses the adequacy of ventilation;

c arterial blood gas (ABG) analysis helps assess the adequacy of ventilation;

d blood glucose only needs to be checked if the patient has a history of diabetes mellitus.

8.2 In acute shortness of breath:

a facemask ventilation should be avoided in a patient whose tracheostomy tube has become dislodged;

b in acute asthma, a rising $PaCO_2$ is a marker of a life-threatening problem;

c a suspected pneumothorax causing tachycardia and hypotension requires an urgent chest X-ray;

d a diagnosis of pulmonary embolus is consistent with finding a sinus tachycardia on the ECG.

8.3 With regard to sepsis:

a hypotension (systolic BP < 90 mmHg) is one of the key diagnostic features;

b fluid resuscitation should be limited to 1500 mL crystalloid (or equivalent volume of colloid);

c the single most important intervention is to give IV antibiotics;

d all patients should be transfused urgently to achieve a haemoglobin of 10 g/dL to improve tissue oxygen delivery.

8.4 Acute kidney injury (AKI):

a is usually classified as pre-renal, intrinsic renal or post renal;

b must have post-renal obstruction excluded in all cases;

c does not occur when the patient has a normal serum creatinine concentration;

d is due to a pre-renal cause when the urine osmolality is increased and the urinary sodium is reduced.

8.5 In the management of cardiac arrhythmias:

a adverse features include a systolic BP <90 mmHg, and syncope;

b a patient with an SVT and no adverse features should be given adenosine as first-line treatment;

c the starting energy for synchronized cardioversion of atrial flutter is 120 J;

d a bradycardia due to complete heart block should be treated initially with 500 µg of atropine.

Answers to short-answer questions

The following answers are only a brief outline. For completeness, further details as in the text indicated should also be included.

Chapter 1

1.1 (*see pages* 4, 5, 8)

By assessing activities of daily living:
- get dressed, distance walked on the flat, stairs climbed, run for a bus.

By estimating how many METs the patient is capable of:
- symptoms when dressing (≤ 2 METs), can garden, walk on the flat (5–7 METS), jogs, play squash (≥ 7 METs).

Perform cardiopulmonary exercise testing:
- measure the patient's anaerobic threshold. If >14 ml/kg/min, no specific risk; <11 ml/kg/min high risk, ITU needed postoperatively.

1.2 (*see page* 7)

- Look at the patient's oro-facial and cervical anatomy.
- Mallampati criteria.
- Thyromental distance.
- Wilson score.
- Calder test.

1.3 (*see page* 12)

I   A healthy patient
II   A patient with a mild to moderate systemic disease process that does not limit the patient's activities in any way
III   A patient with severe systemic disease from any cause that imposes a definite functional limitation on activity
IV   A patient with a severe systemic disease that is a constant threat to life
V   A moribund patient unlikely to survive 24h with or without surgery
VI   A patient declared brain dead whose organs are being removed for transplantation

The patient described would be ASA III; she has systemic illnesses which impose a restriction on her functional activity, but they are not a constant threat to her life at present.

1.4 (*see pages* 8, 9)

This is major surgery. According to the NICE guidelines she will need to have:
- A full blood count (FBC) to identify anaemia (low Hb) and its possible cause (MCV), occult infection (raised WCC), blood clotting problems (low platelet count).

Clinical Anaesthesia Lecture Notes, Fourth Edition. Carl Gwinnutt and Matthew Gwinnutt.
© 2012 John Wiley & Sons, Ltd. Published 2012 by John Wiley & Sons, Ltd.

- Renal function tests (also called urea and electrolytes, U&Es) to identify electrolyte disturbances or impaired renal function as a result of her age, or as a consequence of treatment for hypertension (diuretics, ACEI).
- ECG: to identify cardiac ischaemia, conduction disturbance or arrhythmia, and left ventricular hypertrophy.

In addition she will need:

- Pulmonary function tests to assess the severity of her COPD.
- If dyspnoeic at rest, cyanosed or has a FEV1 <60% predicted, she will need arterial blood gases doing.
- If she has hip pain that makes assessment of exercise tolerance difficult, she may need echocardiography.
- She is unlikely to be able to perform CPEX testing because of her hip if it is very painful.
- She will not need a chest x-ray as this is only required when there are signs or symptoms of pulmonary disease and the patient is to undergo thoracic surgery.

1.5 (*see page* 11)

- *Common (1 in 10 to 1 in 100):* not life threatening and can occur even when anaesthesia has apparently been uneventful. They include; bruising and soreness from the IV cannula, sore throat, headache, dizziness, postoperative nausea and vomiting, retention of urine.
- *Uncommon (1 in 1000):* dental damage, chest infection, an existing condition worsening, awareness during general anaesthesia.
- *Rare (<1 in 10 000):* allergy to the anaesthetic drugs, nerve damage, hypoxic brain injury, death.

Chapter 2

2.1 (*see page* 32)

An LED emits red light, alternating between two different wavelengths in the visible and infrared regions of the electromagnetic spectrum. These are transmitted through, and absorbed by, the tissues, oxyhaemoglobin and deoxyhaemoglobin. Absorption by the tissues is constant while absorption by blood varies with the cardiac cycle. The light reaching the photodetector is converted to an electrical signal, allowing peripheral arterial oxygen saturation (SpO_2) to be calculated.

Limitations:

- it is unreliable; when there is severe vasoconstriction, with certain haemoglobins and when there is excessive movement of the patient;
- it is affected by extraneous light;
- it is not give any indication of the adequacy of alveolar ventilation.

2.2 (*see pages* 24, 25)

- Oxygen is stored in a vacuum-insulated evaporator at −180 °Cs, and at 10–12 bar. The liquid vaporizes and by the time it reaches the operating theatre it is a gas at ambient temperature.
- Nitrous oxide is stored in a bank of cylinders. It is liquid at a pressure of 54 bar. Medical air is supplied either from cylinders or by a compressor.
- All gases are distributed by the piped medical gas and vacuum system and reach the operating theatre at a pressure of 4 bar (medical gas also delivered at 7 bar to power instruments).
- For safety, the hoses are colour coded (oxygen white, nitrous oxide blue and air yellow). They attach to the wall outlets via gas-specific probes and to the anaesthetic machines via non-interchangeable nut and union.

2.3 (*see pages* 25, 26)

The key functions of the anaesthetic machine include:

- accurate control of the flow of gases (oxygen, air, nitrous oxide) via the flowmeters;
- reduction of pressure from any gases supplied from cylinders;
- prevent a hypoxic mixture of gases being delivered to the patient;
- give a warning of oxygen failure;
- add a known concentration of anaesthetic vapour to the gases.

Many modern anaesthetic machines also:

- provide mechanical ventilation for the patient if required;
- monitor the gases and vapours delivered to and expired by the patient;
- scavenge expired and waste gases and vapours.

2.4 (*see pages* 31, 32)

- The pneumatic cuff must have a width that is *40% of the arm circumference* and the internal inflatable bladder should encircle at least half the arm.
- If the cuff is too small, the blood pressure will be overestimated, and if it is too large it will be underestimated.
- The cuff placed around the upper arm is inflated by an electrical pump to a pressure greater than systolic blood pressure.
- The cuff then undergoes controlled deflation.
- A microprocessor-controlled pressure transducer detects variations in cuff pressure resulting from transmitted arterial pulsations.
- Initial pulsations represent systolic blood pressure and peak amplitude of the pulsations equates to mean arterial pressure.
- Diastolic is then calculated using an algorithm.

Chapter 3

3.1 (*see page* 44)

- Suxamethonium molecules enter the neuromuscular junction and compete with Ach, binding to the postsynaptic (nicotinic) receptors on the motor end plate on the muscle membrane.
- Muscle fasciculation is seen as the muscle membrane is depolarized.
- This is followed by paralysis as the suxamethonium molecules remain bound to the receptors keeping the muscle membrane depolarized.
- Recovery occurs spontaneously as suxamethonium is hydrolysed by the enzyme plasma (pseudo-) cholinesterase
- Normal neuromuscular transmission is restored after 4–6 mins.

Side-effects:
- increased intraocular pressure;
- muscular pain;
- histamine release;
- prolonged apnoea in patients with pseudocholinesterase deficiency;
- a significant rise in serum potassium in certain conditions;
- malignant hyperpyrexia;

3.2 (*see page* 49)

They inhibit the enzyme cyclo-oxygenase (COX). This prevents the synthesis of inflammatory mediators (prostaglandins, prostacyclins and thromboxane A2) from arachidonic acids. There are two main isoenzymes of cyclo-oxygenase, COX-1, COX-2. The inhibition of COX-1 produces the unwanted effects, inhibition of COX-2 the desired therapeutic effects.

Relative contraindications	Absolute contraindications
• High risk of intraoperative bleeding e.g. vascular surgery	• Pre-existing renal dysfunction, hyperkalaemia
• Concurrent use of ACE inhibitors, anticoagulants, nephrotoxic drugs	• Cardiac failure
	• Severe hepatic dysfunction
• Hepatic dysfunction	• History of GI bleeding
• Bleeding disorders	• Hypersensitivity to NSAIDs
• Elderly (>65 years)	• Aspirin-induced asthma
• Pregnancy and during lactation	
• Asthma	

3.3 (*see page* 50)

Risk of PONV is associated with:
- female sex;
- being a non-smoker;
- previous history of PONV or motion sickness;
- opioids as part of the anaesthetic technique.

A scoring system that allocates one point for each of the four risk factors listed above has been devised (Apfel score). Patients who score 0 or 1 points are at low risk of PONV, and should not routinely receive anti-emetics. A score of 2 or more points is a high risk of PONV, and patients should receive combination therapy (use drugs with different modes of action).

Drugs that can be used include:
- antihistamines; cyclizine, 50 mg IM or IV;
- 5-hydroxytryptamine antagonists; ondansetron, 4–8 mg orally or IV;
- corticosteroid; dexamethasone, 4–8 mg IV.

3.4 (*see pages* 47,48)

Central effects include:
- analgesia;
- sedation;
- euphoria;
- nausea and vomiting;
- pupillary constriction;
- depression of ventilation.

These can be reversed by naloxone. This has antagonist actions at all the opioid receptors, reversing all the centrally mediated effects of pure opioid agonists.

3.5 (*see pages* 50–53)

A stimulus of sufficient intensity triggers opening of sodium channels. Cell membrane potential increases from −70 mV to +20 mV (action potential). Adjacent voltage-gated sodium channels open, propagating the action potential along the nerve. In myelinated nerves, action potentials can 'jump' between nodes of Ranvier to speed up conduction. The membrane is rapidly repolarized by loss of potassium ions (K^+) from within the cell and by active pumping out of Na^+ in exchange for K^+ by the Na/K pump.

Local anaesthetic drugs work by blocking the sodium channels from within the nerve cell, preventing entry of sodium and subsequent depolarization so that no action potentials can be initiated or propagated.

The relationship between concentration, volume, and dose is given by the formula:

concentration (%) × volume (ml) × 10 = dose (mg), therefore
$$0.75\% \times 15 \times 10 = 112.5 \text{ mg}$$

Toxic dose = 3 mg/kg, max 200 mg without adrenaline
= 6 mg/kg, max 500 mg with adrenaline

Chapter 4

4.1 (*see pages* 62, 63)

Advantages include:
- It avoids repeated attempts at venepuncture in patients with poor veins.

- It avoids venepuncture in an uncooperative child, or patients with needle phobia.
- In patients with airway compromise, it preserves spontaneous ventilation and if airway patency is threatened, further uptake of anaesthetic is prevented, limiting the problem.

Disadvantages include:
- Unconsciousness occurs more slowly than with an IV drug.
- Inhalational drugs are unpleasant to breathe.
- Hypotension and a fall in cardiac output occur with increasing concentrations. This may be difficult to treat until IV access is obtained.
- Hypercapnia (due to respiratory depression) and the vasodilator effect of these drugs lead to increased cerebral blood flow, making this technique unsuitable in patients with raised intracranial pressure.

4.2 (*see pages* 68, 69)

Gold standard:
- measuring carbon dioxide in expired gas (capnometry).

Next best:
- seeing the tracheal tube passing between the vocal cords.

Use an oesophageal detector device:
- fogging on clear plastic tube connectors during expiration.

Less reliable signs are:
- breath sounds on auscultation;
- chest movement on ventilation;
- gurgling sounds over the epigastrium;
- decrease in oxygen saturation (late).

Complications:
- unrecognized oesophageal intubation;
- failed intubation and inability to ventilate the patient;
- failed ventilation after intubation;
- aspiration of regurgitated gastric contents;
- direct trauma to all structures from lips to lungs;
- trauma to adjacent structures during the procedure;
- hypertension and arrhythmias;
- vomiting;
- laryngeal spasm.

4.3 (*see pages* 70, 71)

Infusions of propofol to keep the patient unconscious and an opioid for analgesia (remifentanil, alfentanil). Boluses of fentanyl could also be used or alternatively a regional technique (epidural). A neuromuscular blocking drug will be required for muscle relaxation and ventilation with oxygen-enriched air.

Advantages:
- avoid potential toxic effects of inhalational anaesthetics and use of nitrous oxide;
- improved quality of recovery;
- beneficial in certain types of surgery (neurosurgery);
- reduces pollution.

Disadvantages:
- reliable IV access required;
- risk of awareness if IV infusion fails;
- cost of electronic infusion pumps;
- hypotension.

4.4 (*see pages* 71, 72)

Indications:
- when neuromuscular blocking drugs are used to facilitate surgical access, e.g. laparotomy;
- during thoracotomy to prevent paradoxical movement;
- to prevent unacceptable degree of respiratory depression;
- to allow control of carbon dioxide and cerebral blood flow during neurosurgery;
- whenever a patient needs tracheal intubation for more than a few minutes, e.g. prone surgery, full stomach, shared airway (ENT).

Potential adverse effects:
- there is an increase in ventilation/perfusion (V/Q) mismatch, requiring the use of an increased inspired oxygen concentration;
- reduced venous return to the heart and cardiac output;
- hyperventilation and hypoventilation causing a respiratory alkalosis and a respiratory acidosis respectively with the associated effects on the oxyhaemoglobin dissociation curve;
- excessive tidal volume may cause lung injury;
- reduced systemic and pulmonary blood flow.

4.5 (*see page* 75)

Any deficit the patient has accrued while waiting for surgery.

Intraoperative requirements:
- maintenance fluids during the procedure;
- losses due to surgery; blood, evaporation, third-space losses.

Any vasodilatation secondary to the use of a regional anaesthetic technique.

The volume of fluid required intraoperatively will be:
maintenance fluid: 03:00–10:30, 1.5 mL/kg/h = 900 mL crystalloid;
blood loss 600 mL will require approximately 1500 mL crystalloid;
third-space losses approximately 500 mL;
total approximately 3000 mL.

This does not all have to be given during surgery, normally between 09:00–12:00, i.e. 1000 mL per hour.
If surgery is carried out under spinal anaesthesia, the patient will probably receive an additional 1000 mL in the anaesthetic room to prevent any hypotension associated with vasodilatation.

4.6 (*see pages* 59, 74, 76)

The Surgical Safety Checklist is completed in three stages

Before the induction of anaesthesia ('sign in'):
- Confirm the patient's identity, usually with the patient, their wrist band and case notes.
- Confirm the planned operation, site, and side (if appropriate).
- Check the correct surgical site is clearly marked.
- Check the consent form details are entered correctly and it is signed appropriately by the patient and surgical team.
- Record that the anaesthetic machine has been checked along with the drugs required for the case.
- Check for any known allergies the patient may have.
- Check to ensure that any problems with airway management have been identified.
- Confirm the anticipated blood loss and availability of blood.

Before the start of the surgical intervention (i.e. skin incision or equivalent) ('time out'):
- Confirm that all the team members have introduced themselves by name and role.
- The patient's identity must be confirmed, along with the planned procedure, side and site.
- The anaesthetic, surgical and nursing teams should identify any anticipated problems, e.g. blood loss, equipment issues.

- Antibiotic prophylaxis, glycaemic control and VTE prophylaxis have all been instituted where appropriate.
- Imaging – e.g. X-rays, CT scans – are available and for the correct patient.

Before the team leaves the operating theatre (or at skin closure or its equivalent) ('sign out'):

- Confirmation that all instruments and swabs are complete and accounted for.
- All specimens are correctly labelled.
- The procedure has been recorded accurately.
- Have any equipment issues been identified that need addressing?
- Are there any concerns for the immediate recovery and postoperative management for the patient?

Chapter 5

5.1 (*see page* 79)

- Avoids the systemic effects of drugs used for GA.
- Respiratory depressant drugs avoided.
- There is generally less disturbance of the control of coexisting systemic disease.
- The airway reflexes are preserved.
- May improve surgical access, e.g. during laparotomy.
- Reduced blood loss.
- Can be continued postoperatively to provide pain relief.
- Reduces complications after major surgery.
- A reduction in the equipment required and the cost of anaesthesia.

5.2 (*see page* 84)

- Hypovolaemia may cause severe fall in cardiac output as compensatory vasoconstriction is lost.
- A low, fixed cardiac output, e.g. severe aortic stenosis or heart failure. The reduced venous return further reduces cardiac output, jeopardizing perfusion of vital organs.
- Local skin sepsis risks introducing infection.
- Coagulopathy, anticoagulation and antiplatelet therapy: risks of causing an epidural haematoma. There may also be a small risk in patients taking aspirin and associated drugs which reduce platelet activity. Where heparins are used perioperatively to reduce the risk of deep venous thrombosis, these may be started after the insertion of the epidural or spinal.
- Raised intracranial pressure risks precipitating coning.
- Known allergy to amide local anaesthetic drugs.
- A patient who is totally uncooperative.
- Concurrent disease of the CNS may lead to risk of blame if any subsequent deterioration.
- Previous spinal surgery or abnormal spinal anatomy: may make procedure technically difficult.

5.3 (*see page* 84)

A high spread of the spinal anaesthetic to the thoracic nerves causes progressive sympathetic block, causing vasodilatation and a reduction in venous return to the heart. Cardiac output and blood pressure fall. If the block extends above T5, the cardioaccelerator nerves are also blocked, and the unopposed vagal tone results in a bradycardia. Small falls in blood pressure are tolerated and may be helpful in reducing blood loss.

If the blood pressure falls by >25% of resting value, or the patient becomes symptomatic (see below), treatment consists of:

- oxygen via a facemask;
- IV fluids (crystalloids or colloids) to increase venous return;
- vasopressors to counteract the vasodilatation, either ephedrine, an α- and β-agonist (3 mg IV) or metaraminol, an α-agonist (0.25 mg IV);
- atropine 0.5 mg IV to counteract bradycardia.

5.4 (*see page* 85)

- Mild or early:
  ○ circumoral paraesthesia;
  ○ numbness of the tongue;
  ○ visual disturbances;
  ○ lightheadedness;
  ○ slurred speech;
  ○ twitching;
  ○ restlessness;
  ○ mild hypotension and bradycardia.
- Severe or late:
  ○ grand mal convulsions followed by coma:
  ○ respiratory depression and eventually apnoea;
  ○ cardiovascular collapse with profound hypotension and bradycardia;
  ○ cardiac arrest.

Management:

- Stop giving the local anaesthetic immediately, get help;
- Maintain the airway using basic techniques. Tracheal intubation will be needed if the protective reflexes are absent to protect against aspiration;
- Give oxygen (100%) with support of ventilation if inadequate;
- Raise the patient's legs to encourage venous return and start an IV infusion of crystalloid or colloid. Treat a bradycardia with IV atropine;
- Treat convulsions with diazepam 5–10 mg IV.

If the patient has a cardiac arrest, start lipid emulsion therapy:
give 1.5 mL/kg 20% lipid emulsion (approximately 100 ml) over 1 min;
start an infusion of 20% lipid emulsion at a rate of 15 mL/kg/h.

Chapter 6

6.1 (*see pages* 88, 89)

Factors predisposing to regurgitation and aspiration:
- a full stomach;
- gastric distension following face mask ventilation;
- delayed gastric emptying from any cause (e.g. trauma);
- obstetric patients;
- gastro-oesophageal reflux, hiatus hernia;
- obesity.

Reduction of risks:
- reduction of residual gastric volume;
- increase pH of gastric contents;
- use of cricoid pressure.

6.2 (*see pages* 93, 94)

Clinical signs:
- severe hypotension;
- severe bronchospasm;
- widespread flushing;
- hypoxaemia;
- urticaria;
- angioedema, which may involve the airway;
- pruritus, nausea and vomiting.

Immediate management:
- stop all drugs, call for help;
- maintain a patent airway; give 100% oxygen
- elevate the patient's legs
- give adrenaline, boluses of 0.5 mL of 1:10 000 IV under ECG control; if no ECG is available, give 0.5 mL of 1:1000 IM;
- ensure adequate ventilation;
- start a rapid intravenous infusion of crystalloids 10–20 mL/kg;
- in the absence of a major pulse, start cardiopulmonary resuscitation;
- monitor: ECG, SpO_2, blood pressure, end-tidal CO_2, check the blood gases.

6.3 (*see page* 95)

- An unexplained tachycardia.
- An increased end-tidal CO_2.
- Tachypnoea in spontaneously breathing patients.
- A progressive rise in body temperature.
- Muscle rigidity, failure to relax after suxamethonium, especially persistent masseter spasm.
- Cardiac arrhythmias.
- A falling oxygen saturation and cyanosis.

- Get help.
- Stop all volatile anaesthetic drugs; hyperventilate with 100% oxygen.
- Maintain anaesthesia with total intravenous anaesthetic technique.
- Change the anaesthesia machine and circuits.
- Terminate surgery as soon as practical.
- Monitor core temperature.
- Give dantrolene 2–3 mg/kg IV initially, then 1 mg/kg boluses as required (up to 10 mg/kg may be needed).
- Start active cooling.
- Transfer the patient to the ITU as soon as possible.
- Following an episode, the patient and their family should be referred to a MH unit for investigation of their susceptibility to MH.

6.4 (*see pages* 96–98)

The most important action is to ensure maintenance of oxygenation.
Try insertion of a supraglottic airway device or intubating LMA:
- If successful and oxygenation is maintained, is this airway safe for surgery to proceed? If so, continue.

- If intubation is mandatory for surgery, attempt intubation via SGA or ILM:
  - If successful, continue with surgery.
  - If unsuccessful, wake patient up, postpone surgery.
- If oxygenation cannot be maintained via a SGA or ILM, attempt to ventilate via a facemask:
  - If successful, wake patient up, postpone surgery.
  - If unsuccessful, either reattempt with SGA or perform needle or surgical crico-thyroidotomy depending on skill and equipment.

Chapter 7

7.1 (*see pages* 101–105)

- Hypoventilation: airway obstruction (tongue), respiratory depression (drugs), mechanical impairment (obesity), pulmonary dysfunction (smoking).
- Ventilation/perfusion mismatch: a reduced FRC, development of atelectasis e.g. due to pain, obesity, elderly, upper GI surgery.
- Diffusion hypoxia: use of nitrous oxide

Oxygen masks:
- Hudson mask; 25–60%, flow dependent;
- Hudson with reservoir; up to 85%;
- Nasal catheter; 25–40%;
- Venturi masks; 24–60% depending on which is used.

7.2 (*see pages* 106, 107)

- Hypovolaemia: blood loss, inadequate fluid replacement.
- Cardiac dysfunction: ischaemic heart disease, arrhythmia, valvular heart disease.
- Vasodilatation: sepsis, extensive spread of epidural anaesthesia, anaphylaxis.

Management:
- Ensure adequate oxygenation and ventilation;
- Give IV fluid challenge the volume of which will depend on the patient's blood pressure or known heart failure;
- Observe their response; be prepared to repeat the fluid challenge;
- Get help if there is a poor or no response.

Take blood for:
- FBC, U + Es, cross-match, coagulation screen, blood cultures;
- arterial blood gases analysis, in particular pH, base excess and lactate.

Stop any external haemorrhage with direct pressure. Get surgical assistance if internal haemorrhage is suspected.

If not already done, consider inserting a urinary catheter.

Monitor:
- central venous pressure (CVP);
- 12-lead ECG.

Treat any arrhythmias.

Check extent of epidural action.

May need vasopressors and/or inotropes.

Consider ultrasound to look for free fluid in the chest or abdomen and check cardiac function.

7.3 (*see pages* 108–111)

He will require a minimum of:
Maintenance fluid, 1.5 ml/kg/h water, 1.5 mmol/kg sodium and 1 mmol/L potassium:

$$1.5 \times 80 \times 24 = 2880 \text{ ml water},$$
$$120 \text{ mmol sodium},$$
$$80 \text{ mmol potassium.}$$

In addition, he has signs of hypovolaemia (tachycardia, hypotension, oliguria and feels thirsty), probably as a result of third space losses. This will require an additional 1000 ml fluid (normal saline or Hartmann's).

The losses from the drain will need replacing, 400 ml (saline or Hartmann's).

He is hypokalaemic and hence will need extra potassium (40 mmol).

He is anaemic and will require blood to raise his Hb to 9 g/dL.

Predicted total requirement:
4280 ml, 340 mmol sodium, 120 mmol potassium, 3 units of packed red blood cells.

A number of combinations of fluids could be used. One regime that could be used to achieve this is:
- 1 L 0.9% saline plus 40 mmol KCl over 4 hours;
- 1 L 0.9% saline plus 40 mmol KCl over 4 hours;
- 1 L 4% glucose/0.18% saline plus 40 mmol KCl over 6 hours;
- 1 L 4% glucose/0.18% saline over 6 hours;

- 0.5 L 4% glucose/0.18% saline over 4 hours;
- 3 units PRBC concurrently.

The patient must be reviewed after 6–8 hours to see if there is any change in his status. Early consideration should be given to monitoring his CVP.

7.4 (*see pages* 114, 115)

A PCA device is a microprocessor-controlled syringe pump that can be programmed to deliver a predetermined dose of a drug intravenously when activated by the patient depressing a switch. The maximum dose in any period and any background infusion is predetermined to prevent overdose and, after a dose has been delivered, subsequent doses cannot be given for a preset period – the 'lockout period'. The PCAs record the number of attempts made by the patient to access analgesia, allowing the dose to be adjusted to meet the patient's requirements.

Advantages:
- analgesia matched to the patient's perception of the pain;
- reduced workload for the nursing staff;
- elimination of painful IM injections;
- greater certainty of adequate plasma levels.

Disadvantages:
- expensive to purchase and maintain;
- needs the patient to understand how to use the PCA and be able to trigger the device;
- potential for overdose if incorrectly programmed.

7.5 (*see pages* 117, 118)

Hypotension: Treat acutely with IV fluid and vasopressors. Check the extent of the block; if extensive, reduce the rate of infusion.
Respiratory depression: Treat by supporting ventilation if necessary; stop the epidural infusion; give naloxone according to the severity; seek expert help.
Sedation: Treat by stopping the infusion; if unresponsive or the level of sedation progresses, give naloxone in 0.1 mg increments intravenously; seek expert help.
Pruritus: May respond to antihistamines, atropine or naloxone.
Retention of urine: May require short-term catheterization.

Chapter 8

8.1 (*see pages* 125, 126)

Look for: paradoxical chest and abdominal movements; use of the accessory muscles of respiration, tracheal tug, intercostal recession.
Feel for: movement of air at the patient's mouth.
Listen for: breath sounds at the mouth or nose. Noisy breathing means obstruction.

Management:
- Head tilt, chin lift, suction – reassess.
- Oropharyngeal or nasopharyngeal airway – reassess.
- Give high-flow oxygen.
- If no improvement, call for help urgently, prepare for use of advanced airway.
- If satisfactory, move on to assess adequacy of breathing.

8.2 (*see page* 134)

If not already done, give oxygen 15 L/min via face-mask with reservoir.
Give salbutamol 5 mg via a nebulizer and repeat if no response.
Establish basic monitoring:
- pulse oximetry;
- non-invasive blood pressure;
- ECG (can be monitored via defibrillator pads).

If not done already, get IV access:
- give steroids IV, hydrocortisone 100 mg.

If little or no response:
- give magnesium sulphate, 8 mmol (2 g) slowly IV;
- add inhaled ipratropium 0.5 mg via a nebulizer.

Take an arterial blood sample for blood gas analysis.
Refer to ITU if:
- his PEF worsens despite treatment;
- he is hypoxic, $PaO_2 < 8$ kPa despite treatment;
- he is hypercapnic, $PaCO_2 > 6.0$ kPa, suggesting he is becoming exhausted;
- he is becoming drowsy.

8.3 (*see page* 150)

Confirm cardiac arrest, check for breathing and a central pulse simultaneously.
Restart CPR, ensuring good technique is being used.

Attach self-adhesive defibrillator pads while chest compressions are ongoing.

Plan actions for team members to minimize hands-off time if defibrillation is required.

Stop CPR and check rhythm on monitor, immediately resume CPR. Take less than 10 s.

If VF or VT:
- safely deliver a shock, 150–200 J biphasic;
- without checking rhythm or pulse ensure CPR starts immediately.

Continue CPR for 2 min, after which check the monitor:
- if a rhythm compatible with a cardiac output is seen, check for signs of a circulation, e.g. pulse, increase in ETCO$_2$;
- if VF persists, deliver a second shock, 150–360 J.

After a further 2 min, check the monitor:
- if a rhythm compatible with a cardiac output is seen, check for signs of a circulation;
- if VF persists, deliver a third shock, 150–360 J;
- give 1 mg adrenaline IV and 300 mg amiodarone IV.

Repeat the 2 min sequence of CPR-rhythm check-defibrillation while VF persists.

Give further doses of 1 mg adrenaline every alternate shock, approximately every 3–5 min.

If the patient has a return of spontaneous circulation (ROSC), organize post-resuscitation care. This will require transfer of the patient to a critical care area.

If PEA or asystole:
- Give adrenaline 1 mg IV.

After 2 min check rhythm. If organized electrical activity is seen, check for signs of circulation:
- if there is ROSC, organize post-resuscitation care;
- if there is no ROSC, continue CPR for 2 min, give further doses of adrenaline every 3–5 min;
- recheck the rhythm check every 2 min;
- if there is a change to VF/VT at the rhythm check, change to the shockable side of the algorithm.

While CPR is ongoing, identify and treat any reversible causes (4Hs & 4Ts)

8.4 (*see pages* 143, 144)

- Hypotension.
- Pyrexia.

- Tachycardia.
- Warm, flushed peripheries with normal capillary refill time (CRT).
- A bounding pulse with a wide pulse pressure.
- Oliguria.
- May be confused.

Management:
- give oxygen 15 L/min via facemask with reservoir;
- get large-bore IV access; take bloods for FBC, U + Es, blood glucose, CRP, coagulation screen, blood cultures;
- give a fluid challenge, 20 ml/kg crystalloid or equivalent volume of colloid over 10–15 min, maintain MAP >65 mmHg;
- give IV broad-spectrum antibiotics;
- at the same time start monitoring with ECG, NIBP, pulse oximetry;
- take an arterial blood sample and measure serum lactate to assess the severity of septic shock;
- get help;
- order a CXR, abdominal ultrasound or CT to try and identify source of sepsis;
- send stool sample if diarrhoea.

If hypotension doesn't respond to fluid resuscitation, vasopressors may be required. This will require transfer to ITU for invasive haemodynamic monitoring

8.5 (*see pages* 145, 146)

Immediate management:
- Perform an ABCDE assessment and at the same time attach ECG, non-invasive BP, pulse oximeter.
- Ask the patient how he or she is.

A: Check that the airway is patent; look for chest movement, listen for sounds of air movement and any associated abnormal noises and feel for air movement:
- if the airway is patent give oxygen 15 L/min via facemask with reservoir;
- if the airway is not patent, use basic manoeuvres and reassess, get help urgently.

B: Look for use of the accessory muscles of respiration, tracheal tug, abdominal breathing, sweating, central cyanosis. Count the respiratory rate. Look at the depth of each breath and symmetry of movement of the two sides of the chest. Auscultate the chest. Feel for; the position of the trachea in the suprasternal notch, equality of expansion and finally percussion of both sides.

- If the breathing is adequate, check the SpO_2 and adjust the oxygen to give a value of 94–98%. If the patient is known to have severe COPD, adjust to 88–92%.
- If the breathing is inadequate, start ventilation using a bag-mask and call cardiac arrest team.

C: Look at; the colour of the hands and digits and at the state of the peripheral veins. Measure the CRT. Look for signs of blood or ECF loss; from bleeding from the wound or into drains, nasogastric or other loss. Auscultate the heart and feel both peripheral and central pulses. Measure the blood pressure:

- if it has not been done already, get IV access, take bloods and start a fluid challenge depending on the patient's blood pressure;
- check that the urinary catheter is patent and not leaking;
- organize for an ABG to be taken.

D: Assess the level of consciousness using the GCS and examine the pupils.

- Check the patient's drug chart.

E: A full head-to-toe, front and back examination. Concentrate on the most relevant areas, in this case the wound and then abdomen.

Review the patient's notes and charts. Assimilate the data on charts by systematic analysis. Study both absolute values of vital signs and their trends. Check that important routine medications are prescribed and being administered. Look for potential interactions. Review the results of all laboratory and radiological investigations.

Summon senior help and, while waiting for this to arrive, reassess the patient using the ABCDE approach to identify the cause.

The most likely cause is inadequate fluid intake as a result of:

- losses from drains, gastrointestinal tract (vomiting, diarrhoea, fistulae);
- third-space losses after major surgery;
- haemorrhage;
- sepsis.

8.6 (*see pages* 147, 148)

The most likely diagnosis is that he is suffering from an acute coronary syndrome (ACS).

Initial treatment will consist of:

- aspirin, 300 mg orally, crushed or chewed;
- nitrates, usually sublingual GTN, unless very hypotensive;
- oxygen titrated to a SpO_2 94–98%;
- analgesia, usually IV diamorphine, titrated to relieve pain;
- attach to a monitor (can use defibrillator pads).

Send bloods for FBS, U+Es, glucose, cardiac troponins.

Order a 12-lead ECG.

Contact cardiologists.

If the ECG confirms an ACS, give low molecular weight heparin or fondaparinux, subcutaneously, in a therapeutic dose.

Start clopidogrel, if no contraindication.

If not contraindicated, a beta-blocker should be given and a statin.

If the ECG confirms STEMI, consider primary percutaneous coronary intervention (PCI) or fibrinolytic therapy.

Answers to true/false questions

Chapter 1

1.1

A 49-year old woman is seen in the preop clinic, prior to having a laparoscopic cholecystectomy. She has a BMI = 39 kg/m², type 2 diabetes and hypertension. She is currently taking metformin, ramipril, aspirin and simvastatin. She will require the following investigations:

a T: She is diabetic, hypertensive and obese, all of which increase the risk of ischaemic heart disease.

b F: She does not meet any of the criteria for requiring a CXR.

c T: Diabetes may impair renal function affecting both her FBC and U + Es.

d F: She does not have a history of coagulopathy, and is not on warfarin. Low-dose aspirin does not necessitate a coagulation screen.

1.2

Difficulty with tracheal intubation is suggested by finding:

a F: <7 cm suggests difficulty.

b T: This is Mallampati grade III, which suggests difficulty.

c F: This does not suggest a reduced view at laryngoscopy.

d T: An increased BMI suggests difficulty with intubation.

1.3

The following are common risks (1:10 to 1:100) of anaesthesia:

a T: The risk can be stratified using the Apfel score.

b T: A common side effect of opioids, anticholinergics, and neuraxial blockade.

c F: Occurs approximately in 1 in 1000 cases.

d F: Occurs in less than 1 in 10 000 cases.

1.4

The following factors increase the risk of VTE:

a F: Age >60 years increases the risk.

b T: Obesity increases the risk.

c T: As well as those taking oestrogen containing oral contraceptive pills.

d T: The risk is significantly higher until approximately 30 days after surgery.

1.5

In the assessment of the cardiovascular system:

a T: Anaesthesia and surgery with a blood pressure this high risks serious complications such as perioperative myocardial infarction or stroke.

b T: Echocardiography can be used to assess heart valve anatomy, function and pressure gradients across the valves.

c T: Dobutamine can be given to raise heart rate and contractility, simulating exercise while an echo is being performed to assess the ventricular muscle's response.

Clinical Anaesthesia Lecture Notes, Fourth Edition. Carl Gwinnutt and Matthew Gwinnutt.
© 2012 John Wiley & Sons, Ltd. Published 2012 by John Wiley & Sons, Ltd.

d F: Cardiopulmonary exercise (CPX) testing assesses the body's ability to increase oxygen delivery to tissues to meet demand.

Chapter 2

2.1

When using a circle anaesthetic breathing system:
a F: CO_2 is absorbed by the soda lime.
b T: Oxygen and vapour in the circuit are rebreathed.
c F: Absorption of anaesthetic by the patient and fresh gas flow will affect the concentration in the circle and therefore it must be monitored independently.
d F: A circle can be used both for spontaneous and controlled ventilation.

2.2

Oximeters
a F: They become increasingly unreliable below an SpO_2 of 90%.
b F: They give no indication of ventilation as hypoventilation can be compensated for by increasing the inspired oxygen concentration.
c T: This is what they are measuring but they are most accurate above a SpO_2 of 90%.
d F: They overestimate saturation in the presence of carboxyhaemoglobin and underestimate in the presence of methaemoglobin.

2.3

Capnometers
a F: It absorbs infrared light.
b F: It is lower, in health by 0.7 kPa or 5 mmHg, but can increase in the presence of certain diseases, such as COPD.
c T: Is inversely proportional to alveolar ventilation.
d F: The gap between arterial and end-tidal carbon dioxide increases (end-tidal falls), mainly due to the development of increased areas of ventilation/perfusion mismatch.

2.4

Medical gases
a F: It is supplied at a pressure of 400 kPa or 4 bar.

b F: The pipelines carrying N_2O are coloured blue.
c F: They only control flow, not pressure.
d T: At room temperature nitrous oxide becomes a liquid when it is under high pressure, unlike oxygen, which is always a gas at room temperature.

2.5

Supra-glottic airway devices
a F: As they sit above the larynx, they do not isolate and seal the airway. This is only achieved by a cuffed tracheal tube.
b F: They can be used to provide positive pressure ventilation provided the airway pressures are kept reasonably low (<25 cmH$_2$O).
c F: Only the i-gel$^®$ has a moulded gel cuff, others have an inflatable cuff.
d F: There are a wide range of sizes available, suitable for neonates weighing <5 kg upwards.

Chapter 3

3.1

Using an IV drug to induce anaesthesia
a T: As does thiopentone.
b F: This is why it can be used as an infusion for TIVA.
c F: Thiopentone induces anaesthesia very smoothly; these effects are seen with etomidate.
d F: Ketamine causes profound analgesia.

3.2

Suxamethonium
a F: It is the only depolarizing neuromuscular blocking drug.
b T: This is why it is used for RSI.
c F: It cannot be reversed; recovery occurs after metabolism by pseudocholinesterase.
d F: It causes an increase in plasma potassium, which can be life-threatening in some conditions.

3.3

Local anaesthetic drugs
a F: They enter the nerves in the unionized form but it is the ionized form that blocks sodium channels.

b T: Small diameter nerves are blocked before large ones.
c T: Bupivacaine is particularly cardiotoxic.
d F: The maximum safe dose is 3 mg/kg. This is the dose with adrenaline.

3.4

Morphine
a T: NSAIDs are more effective for treating pain from bone and soft tissue injuries.
b F: The peak effect occurs in 5 to 10 min.
c F: It is a Schedule 2 drug.
d F: It causes pupillary constriction (miosis) due to its action on the Edinger–Westphal nucleus.

3.5

Inhalational anaesthesia
a F: Nitrous oxide is not very potent and to prevent hypoxia it is only feasible to give 70% N_2O with 30% O_2. This is an insufficient concentration to ensure reliably adequate depth of anaesthesia for surgery.
b T: It allows comparison of the alveolar concentrations of various anaesthetic drugs needed to achieve the same depth of anaesthesia.
c F: The more soluble the drug, the more readily it dissolves in the blood, and it takes longer for the partial pressure of the drug to rise to a level which causes anaesthesia.
d F: It is irritant to the airways when high concentrations are given resulting in salivation and coughing, and it is relatively soluble in blood making it relatively slow in onset.

Chapter 4

4.1

The following are essential monitors during anaesthesia:
a T: Provides information about heart rate, rhythm and any ischaemia.
b T: Non-invasive blood pressure measurement is one of the essential monitors during anaesthesia, in more complex situations invasive arterial blood pressure measurement will be needed.
c F: Only required if surgery lasts longer than 30 min.

d T: This device has been shown to reduce significantly the incidence of adverse events during anaesthesia

4.2

Oesophageal intubation can be confirmed rapidly using:
a F: A decrease in oxygen saturation detected by pulse oximetry occurs late, particularly if the patient has been preoxygenated.
b T: Carbon dioxide ($> 0.2\%$) indicates the tube is in the airway but does not indicate when the tube has been inserted too far and lies in a main bronchus.
c F: These can be transmitted from the oesophagus, particularly if listening anteriorly.
d T: But only if a good view of the cords is obtained.

4.3

During general anaesthesia:
a F: Theoretically there is no time limit for how long a patient can breathe spontaneously.
b T: Due to the loss of chest-wall muscle tone and the abdominal contents pushing the diaphragm into the chest.
c T: This requires an increase in the oxygen concentration to compensate.
d F: Venous return is impeded and cardiac output reduced.

4.4

Intraoperatively
a T: Particularly during prolonged procedures.
b T: But will need to be increased if the patient is pyrexial.
c F: Most patients will need blood when they have lost $> 30\%$ of their blood volume.
d F: It may cause hyperchloraemic acidosis.

4.5

When positioning the patient for surgery:
a F: It is the ulnar nerve that lies posterior to the medial epicondyle of the humerus and can be damaged here.
b T: So care must be taken to keep the head in a neutral position.
c T: To avoid traction on the brachial plexus. If both arms are abducted the head should be kept in a central position.
d F: In the Trendelenberg position, gravity causes the abdominal contents move

towards the thorax and compromises ventilation.

Chapter 5

5.1

Regional anaesthesia:
a F: Spontaneous ventilation can be preserved and respiratory depressant drugs avoided.
b F: Blood loss may actually be decreased.
c T: There is less disturbance partly due to a modification of the stress response.
d F: Muscle relaxation and contraction of the bowel may improve access.

5.2

Local anaesthetic drugs
a F: This would be dangerous. They can be used IV after application of a tourniquet (Bier's block).
b F: This would cause nerve damage. They must only be injected adjacent to nerves.
c T: This is a common use, for example in suturing lacerations.
d T: This is spinal anaesthesia.

5.3

When performing epidural anaesthesia:
a F: As the epidural space extends from the craniocervical junction at C1 to the sacrococcygeal membrane and anaesthesia can theoretically be safely instituted at any level in between.
b F: This would indicate the needle has been inserted too far and is the technique used for spinal anaesthesia.
c F: The volume injected is one of the main determinants of spread.
d T: The addition of opioids improves the quality and duration of analgesia.

5.4

Contraindications to performing spinal anaesthesia include:
a T: This risks causing an epidural haematoma.
b T: The low fixed cardiac output will be further reduced by the vasodilatation and reduced venous return.
c T: Risk of introducing infection and causing meningitis or ventriculitis.

d T: These patients are likely to be hypovolaemic and very vasoconstricted. Any sudden vasodilatation would cause massive fall in blood pressure and cardiac output.

5.5

Local anaesthetic toxicity
a T: If injected into a vascular area or inadvertently directly IV.
b T: Convulsions may be the first sign of a massive overdose.
c F: Initial treatment would be to stop if still injecting and then use an ABC approach, so ensuring a patent airway and giving oxygen would take priority.
d F: Systemic toxicity with epidural anaesthesia is rare (< 1 in 10 000 patients).

Chapter 6

6.1

Cricoid pressure
a F: It is to prevent passive regurgitation of gastric contents.
b T: It is the only complete cartilaginous ring in the larynx and anterior force is transmitted back onto the oesophagus, which lies anterior to the bodies of the lower cervical vertebra.
c T: Gentle application (10 N) before induction, increasing (to 30 N) as the patient loses consciousness.
d F: Should only be released upon the anaesthetist's request, once the tracheal tube is confirmed as being in the trachea.

6.2

When anaesthetising a patient for a caesarean section:
a F: There are a number of increased risks associated with general anaesthesia. It is not the preferred choice of technique.
b T: Due to a relaxed lower oesophageal sphincter and mechanical compression of the stomach by the gravid uterus.
c T: Abolition of the sympathetic outflow from the spinal cord leads to profound vasodilatation and hypotension within minutes of performing the spinal. Vasopressors must be ready prepared to allow prompt treatment.

d F: A tilt of 10 to 15° to the left is needed to prevent aortocaval compression by the gravid uterus. Obviously care needs to be taken to ensure the patient does not fall off of the operating table.

6.3

One lung ventilation

a T: Collapse of one lung allows surgical access to the mediastinum, thoracic spine or the lung.

b T: It can be left or right-sided depending on which main bronchus the bronchial limb is designed to enter.

c F: A right-sided tube is more likely to obstruct the right upper lobe bronchus.

d T: There is a significant shunt due to blood perfusing the unventilated lung.

6.4

In the management of anaphylaxis:

a F: Adrenaline is the single most important treatment.

b F: The dose of adrenaline is 0.5 mL of 1 in 1000 IM, or if there is ECG monitoring available 0.5 mL of 1 in 10 000 IV can be given.

c F: Intubation may be difficult due to laryngeal oedema.

d T: The haemodynamic instability may persist and there may also be a second exacerbation.

6.5

In the management of malignant hyperthermia:

a T: Any volatile drug must be stopped and the patient will become aware if an alternative method of anaesthesia is not maintained. Propofol is safe to give in MH.

b F: This is not always possible. Surgery should be completed as quickly and as safely as possible.

c F: Dantrolene is the only specific treatment for MH. Whilst MH is due to a problem with calcium release, verapamil has no effect.

d T: Skeletal muscle is broken down releasing potassium and myoglobin, which can cause hyperkalaemia and AKI.

Chapter 7

7.1

Ventilation/perfusion mismatch:

a T: Also if there is a reduced cardiac output, as this causes reduced perfusion of the lungs.

b T: V/Q > 1 results in ventilation but no perfusion and so is wasted ventilation or dead space.

c T: V/Q = 0 results in perfusion but no ventilation and so deoxygenated blood is effectively shunted straight back into the systemic circulation.

d T: As well as smokers, those with pre-existing lung disease, and following upper abdominal and thoracic surgery.

7.2

Under normal circumstances:

a T: The remaining 1/3 is extracellular and split between interstitial (2/3) and intravascular (1/3).

b F: This is double what is required.

c F: 2000 mL of sodium chloride contains 308 mmol of both sodium and chloride, far in excess of what is needed.

d T: In addition 0.1–0.2 mmol/kg of calcium, magnesium and phosphate.

7.3

The following are features of the stress response following major surgery:

a F: ADH production is increased.

b T: Aldosterone levels rise, as do levels of rennin, angiotensin, and cortisol.

c F: Increased ADH and aldosterone result in sodium and water retention by the kidneys and urine output falls.

d F: Not if careful thought is given to fluid balance and renal perfusion.

7.4

Postoperative analgesia

a T: Patients' perceptions of pain, and their response to analgesics are both very variable.

b T: By allowing improved coughing and reducing respiratory complications, improved mobility and reduced risk of VTE.

c F: Multi-modal regimes achieve better analgesia and often allow lower doses of each drug to be given thereby reducing adverse effects.

d F: Active metabolites can accumulate, the pump can be programmed incorrectly, others can press it on the patient's behalf.

7.5

Complications of epidural
  a T: Due to a fall in blood pressure and relative hypovolaemia.
  b T: A side effect of opioids.
  c T: Due to accidental dural puncture.
  d T: May be due to excessive doses of local anaesthetic but there must be a high index of suspicion of epidural haematomas or abscesses causing cord compromise.

Chapter 8

8.1

During the initial assessment of an acutely unwell adult patient:
  a F: Abnormalities should be treated at each stage of the assessment before moving on.
  b F: It is possible to have a normal SpO_2 with inadequate ventilation and consequent hypercarbia.
  c T: An ABG will measure the $PaCO_2$, which is inversely related to ventilation.
  d F: All acutely unwell patients should have a blood glucose checked, especially those with a low GCS.

8.2

In acute shortness of breath:
  a F: Patients with a tracheostomy usually have a patent upper airway, therefore facemask ventilation, with the hole in the neck covered, is appropriate.
  b T: This is a sign that the patient is tiring and usually signifies the need for ventilatory support.
  c F: Delay to obtain a chest x-ray may mean the patient deteriorates to the point of cardiac arrest. In this situation, immediate needle decompression is needed.
  d T: Other rarer ECG changes include S1, Q3 and T3 patterns, and signs of right heart strain.

8.3

Sepsis:
  a F: This is not one of the four diagnostic criteria for SIRS/sepsis, however if present despite fluid resuscitation it does help define septic shock.
  b F: Initial fluid resuscitation should be 20 mL/kg crystalloid; 1500 mL would be the starting volume for a 75 kg patient, not the maximum volume.
  c T: These should be given immediately after blood cultures have been obtained, within 3 hours of new admission, and within 1 hour for inpatients.
  d F: This is not one of the 6 h bundle and has no evidence.

8.4

Acute kidney injury:
  a T: Pre-renal is the most common cause in the postoperative period.
  b T: As this is easily treated.
  c F: GFR can drop from 125 mL/min to only 30 mL/min before any rise in creatinine is seen.
  d T: This shows the kidney is trying and able, to retain sodium and concentrate the urine, which it does in response to poor perfusion – i.e. a pre-renal cause.

8.5

In the management of cardiac arrhythmias:
  a T: Other signs include heart failure and myocardial ischaemia.
  b F: Vagal manoeuvres should be tried first, followed by adenosine if these don't work.
  c T: A lower energy (70 J) is used for atrial flutter.
  d T: Regardless of whether adverse features are present or not as the risk of deterioration to cardiac arrest is high. Expert help will also be needed as the patient may need temporary or permanent pacing.

Index

Page numbers in *italics* denote figures, those in **bold** denote tables.

ABCDE system   125–30
Acute Illness Management (AIM)   122
acute kidney injury   **145**
Acute Life-threatening Event Recognition and
        Treatment (ALERT)   122
acutely ill patients   121–58
    assessment   121–2, 124–30
        airway   125–6, **126**
        breathing   126–8, **127**
        circulation   128–9, **129**
        disability   129–30, **129**
        exposure/examination   130
    clinical scoring systems   122–3, **123**
    critical care outreach team   123, **124**
    deterioration in   131
    emergency management   131–57
        see also specific conditions
    further actions   130–1
    initial approach to patient   125
    receiving a call   123–4
    recognition   121–2
adrenaline (epinephrine)   52, 94
Advanced Life Support (ALS)   122
Advanced Paediatric Life Support (APLS)   122
Advanced Trauma Life Support (ATLS)   122
adverse drug reactions
    anaphylaxis   93–4
    suxamethonium   44
air, medical   25
    cylinder colour   **24**
    see also anaesthetic gases
Airtraq   23, *23*
airway   63–69, *63, 64*
    assessment   6–8, *7, 8*, 125–6, **126**
    nasopharyngeal   19, *19*, 64–5, *65*
    noises   **126**
    obstruction *see* airway obstruction
    oropharyngeal   19, *19*, 63–4, *64*
    problems   65
    see also airway equipment; tracheal intubation
airway equipment   18–24, 100
    adjuncts   19
    facemasks   18–19, *19*, 65, *65*
    laryngoscopes   22–4, 67
    see also supraglottic airway devices

airway obstruction   102, **126**
    lower airway problems, acute   134, 137–41
        asthma   134, 137
        pneumonia   137
        pneumothorax   138
        pulmonary embolism   140–1, *140*
        pulmonary oedema   139–40, **139**, *140*
    upper airway   132–4
        blocked tracheostomy   133–4
        external compression post-surgery   133
        reduced consciousness level   132
        swelling/tumour   132–3
        treatment   133
albumin   **55**
alcohol intake   6
alfentanil   **47**
allergies   5, 94
    latex   94
    see also anaphylaxis
alveolar hypoventilation   101–3, *102*
amethocaine   51
    risk indicators   12–13, **12**
    risks   11–12
    safe delivery   24–31
    total intravenous   44
anaesthetic drugs
    inhaled   42–3, **42**
    intravenous   40–1, **41**
    see also individual drugs
anaesthetic assessment   3–8
    drug history and allergies   5
    exercise tolerance   4–5
    family history   5
    investigations   8–11
    medical history   3–4
    physical examination   6–8
    previous anaesthetics/operations   5
    social history   5–6
anaesthetic gases   24–5
    cylinder colours   **24**
    flow control   25–6, *25*
    medical air   25
    nitrous oxide   24–5, 42, 43
    oxygen   24
    pollution   29–30

Clinical Anaesthesia Lecture Notes, Fourth Edition. Carl Gwinnutt and Matthew Gwinnutt.
© 2012 John Wiley & Sons, Ltd. Published 2012 by John Wiley & Sons, Ltd.

anaesthetic machines   25, *25*, 29, *29*
    preoperative check   58
anaesthetic record   76
anaesthetic vapours   26, *26*
analgesia
    combined techniques   119
    infiltration   80–1, *80*
    NSAIDs   40, 49, **49**
    opioids   46–9, **47**, 113, **115**
    paracetamol   40, 49
    patient-controlled   114–15
    postoperative pain   112–19
    premedication   40
    sites of action   *114*
    see also regional anaesthesia
analgesic drugs   46–9
anaphylaxis   93–4
    causes   94
    investigations   94
    management   94
angina   147
anti-emetics   40, 50, **50**
antibiotics
    allergy   94
    premedication   40
anticholinesterases   45–6
anticoagulants, prophylactic   40
antidiuretic hormone (ADH)   111
antihistamines   94
anuria   106, 145
    see also oliguria
aortocaval compression   90–1
Apfel score   50
arrhythmias   149–50
    bradycardias   107, 150
    postoperative   106–7
    tachycardias   107, 149–50
    and tracheal intubation   69
arterial blood gases
    pneumonia   137
    pulmonary embolism   140
arterial cannulation   62
ASA physical status scale   **12**
aspiration   69, 92–3
    at induction   92–3
    management   92–3
    reducing risks of   88–9, *89*
    with supra-glottic airway   93
aspiration pneumonia   137
asthma   134
    treatment   134
atracurium   **45**
AVPU   **123**

basilic vein   60
bispectral index (BIS)   36
blood glucose   8
blood loss   36

blood pressure   **123**
    invasive/direct monitoring   34, **143**
    non-invasive monitoring   31–2
blood/blood components   55–6
    predepositing   56
    risk of transfusion   55–6
brachial plexus block   81
bradycardias   150
    central neural blockade   84
    postoperative   107
breathing   126–8, **127**
    abnormal   126–7
    rate   **123**
breathing systems   26–8
    circle system   27–8, *27*
    components of   26–7
    mechanical ventilation   28
    monitoring   36
breathlessness *see* dyspnoea
bronchodilators   94
Buccastem   *109*
bupivacaine   52, **53**
buprenorphine   48
BURP manoeuvre   96

caesarean section   89–91
Calder test   7
cannulas, intravascular   30, *30*
capillary refill time   129
capnometry   33, **33**, 67
carbon dioxide
    cylinder colour   **24**
    $PaCO_2$ *102*, 128
cardiac arrest   150–3, *151*, *152*
cardiac arrhythmias *see* arrhythmias
cardiac output
    and hypotension   106–7
    low   84
    and mechanical ventilation   103
    oesophageal Doppler monitoring   34–5, *35*
    pulse analysis monitoring   35, *35*
cardiogenic shock   144–5
    investigations   145
    treatment   144–5
cardiopulmonary exercise (CPX) testing   8–9, **9**
cardiopulmonary resuscitation (CPR)   *152*
cardiovascular disease, medical referral   9
cardiovascular system
    history   3–4, **4**
    obese patients   10
    physical examination   6
Care of the Critically Ill Surgical Patient (CCrISP)   122
catheter over needle technique   61
cell savers   31, 56
central neural blockade   80
    complications   84–5, **84**
        hypotension and bradycardia   84
        nausea and vomiting   84–5

post-dural puncture headache   85
epidural anaesthesia   81–3, *82*, 84
spinal anaesthesia   83–4, *83*
central respiratory depression   102
central venous cannulation   60–1, *61*
    equipment   61
    internal jugular vein   60–1, **61**
    subclavian vein   61
central venous pressure   34, **34**, 111
cephalic vein   60
cerebral haemorrhage   102
cerebral ischaemia   102
cervical spine X-ray   8
chest movement   125–6
chest pain   147–9
    angina   147
    myocardial infarction   3, 148–9, *148*
chest X-ray   8
    cardiogenic shock   145
    pneumonia   137
    pulmonary oedema   *140*
chlorphenamine   94
circle system   27–8, *27*
circulation
    assessment   128–9, **129**
    collapse   85–6, 93
cisatracurium   **45**
clinical scoring systems   122–3, **123**
coagulation screen   8
coagulopathy   84
cocaine   51
colloids   54–5, **55**
coma   129–30, **130**
    see also unconscious patients
community-acquired pneumonia   137
conscious level, decreased   **129**, 154–7
COX-1 inhibitors   49
COX-2 inhibitors   49
cricoid pressure   89, *89*
critical care outreach team   123, **124**
cryoprecipitate   55
crystalloids   53–4, **54**
cyclizine   **50**, *109*

dantrolene   95, 100
desflurane   **42**
dexamethasone   **50**, *109*
diabetes mellitus   5
diaphragmatic splinting   102
diffusion hypoxia   104
disability   129–30, **129**
dorsal metacarpal vein   60
dose calculation   53
drugs   39–57
    dose calculation   53
    history of use   5
    see also specific drugs and classes
dyspnoea   132–41

Early Warning Score (EWS)   122, **123**
ECG   8, 31
    pulmonary embolism   141
    pulmonary oedema   139
echocardiography   9
    transthoracic   143
electrocardiogram *see* ECG
electrolytes   8
emergence from anaesthesia   76–7
emergency surgery   88
EMLA   40
endocrine disorders, medical
        referral   10
entonox
    cylinder colour   **24**
    postoperative analgesia   119
epidural anaesthesia   81–3, *82*
    caesarean section   90
    complications   117–19
        post-dural puncture headache   85,
        118–19
    contraindications   84
    inadequate   118
    postoperative   116–17
epinephrine *see* adrenaline
Epworth sleepiness assessment   **11**
equipment
    airway *see* airway equipment
    cell savers   31
    giving sets and fluid warmers   30
    intravascular cannulas   30, *30*
    monitoring   36
    patient warming   30–1
    postanaesthesia care unit   100–1
    syringe pumps   31
    tracheal intubation   67
    ultrasound   31
etomidate   **41**
European Trauma Course (ETC)   122
eutectic mixture of local anaesthetics
        see EMLA
exercise tolerance   4–5

facemasks   18–19, *19*, 65, *65*
    oxygen delivery   104–5, *105*
failed intubation   96–8
family history   5
fentanyl   **47**, 113
fibreoptic bronchoscope   23, *23*
flowmeters   25–6, *25*
fluid therapy   108–11
    clinical assessment   111
    major surgery   110–11
    minor surgery   108–10
    monitoring   111
    stress response   111
    third space losses   110–11
fluid warmers   30

fluids 53–6
  colloids 54–5, **55**
  crystalloids 53–4, **54**
  intraoperative 75–6
    accrued deficit 75
    requirements 75–6
  see also blood/blood components
fondiparinux 14
fresh frozen plasma 55
functional residual capacity 103

gastric contents
  aspiration *see* aspiration
  full stomach 88
  pH/volume 39–40, 89
gastric emptying, delayed 88
gastrointestinal system, obese patients 11
Gelofusine **55**
general anaesthesia 58–78
  airway 63–70
  emergence from 76–7
  induction 62–3
  maintenance 70–2
  preoperative checks 58–9
  preparation for 59–62
  transfer to operating theatre 72–6
giving sets 30
Glasgow Coma Scale **130**
glyceryl trinitrate (GTN), transdermal 40
gum elastic bougie 24

haemaccel **55**
haematological disorders, medical referral 10
haemodilution, preoperative 56
haemothorax 103
Hartmann's solution **54**
heart failure 3, **4**
helium/oxygen, cylinder colours **24**
heparin 14
hetastarch **55**
hiatus hernia 5
high airflow with oxygen enrichment 105, *105*
hormone replacement therapy 5
hospital-acquired pneumonia 137
Hudson mask 105, *105*
hydrocortisone 94
hyoscine **50**
hyperpyrexia, malignant 95
hypertension 3–4
  postoperative 108
  and tracheal intubation 69
hypoglycaemia 154–5
  investigations 154–155
  treatment 154
hypopnoea syndrome 10–11
hypotension 141–5
  causes **129**
    cardiogenic shock 144–5

    central neural blockade 84, 117
    hypovolaemic shock 84, 106, 142–3
    sepsis/septic shock 143–4
  postoperative 106–7
hypothermia 103
hypovolaemia/hypovolaemic shock 106,
  142–3, 157
  investigations 143
  treatment 142–3
hypoxaemia 101–4, 157
  alveolar hypoventilation 101–3, *102*
  diffusion hypoxia 104
  management 104–6, *105*
  pulmonary diffusion defects 104
  reduced inspired oxygen concentration 104
  ventilation-perfusion mismatch 103–4, **104**
hypoxia
  diffusion 104
  oesophageal intubation 69
    aspiration
    failed intubation

induction of anaesthesia 62–3
  aspiration during 92–3
  rapid sequence 89
infiltration analgesia 80–1, *80*
informed consent 14–16
  definition 14
  evidence of 16
  obtaining 15–16
  patient information 14–15
  unconscious patients 16
inhalational anaesthesia 42–3, **42**
  maintenance 70
  minimum alveolar concentration 43, **43**
  solubility 42–3
internal jugular vein, cannulation 60–1, **61**
intracranial haemorrhage 155–6, *155*
intracranial pressure, raised 84
intrathecal anaesthesia *see* spinal anaesthesia
intravascular cannulas 30, *30*
intravenous access 60–2
  arterial cannulation 62
  central venous cannulation 60–1, *61*
  complications **60**
intravenous anaesthetic drugs 40–1, **41**
  total *see* total intravenous anaesthesia
intubating laryngeal mask airway 20,
  20, 21
intubation *see* tracheal intubation
investigations 2, 8–11
  see also individual investigations and tests
ipratropium 94
isoflurane **42**

jaundice 5

ketamine **41**

laryngeal mask airway (LMA) 19–20, *20*
  intubating 20, *20, 21*
laryngeal spasm 69
laryngectomy *136*
laryngoscopes 22–4, 67
  direct 22, *22*
  gum elastic bougie 24
  indirect 22–3, *22, 23*
lateral position 73, *73*
latex allergy 94
left ventricular dysfunction 106
leg weakness 118
levobupivacaine **53**
lidocaine 52, **53**
  infiltration analgesia 80–1
lipid emulsions 100
lithotomy position 73
liver function tests 8
Lloyd-Davies position 73
local anaesthesia *see* regional anaesthesia
local anaesthesia
  role of 79–80
  technique 80, *81*
local anaesthetic agents 50–3, **53**
  mechanism of action 50–1
  overdose 85
  toxicity 85–6
    circulatory collapse 85–6
    management of 85–86
  see also individual drugs
loss of consciousness *see* consciousness, reduced
low urine output 145–147
  investigations 146–147
  treatment 146

magnesium 94
maintenance of anaesthesia 70–2
  inhalational anaesthesia 70
  total intravenous anaesthesia 70–1
malignant hyperpyrexia
presentation 95
  anaesthesia for susceptible patients 95
  immediate management 95
  investigation of family 95
Mallampati criteria 7, *7*
mechanical ventilation 28, 71–2, 77
  and cardiac output 103
medical history 3–4
  cardiovascular system 3–4, **4**
  respiratory system 4
medical referral 9–10
metabolic disorders, obese patients 11
metoclopramide 40, **50**
midazolam **41**
minimum alveolar concentration (MAC) 43, **43**
Misuse of Drugs Act (1971) 48
Misuse of Drugs Regulations (2001) 48
mivacurium **45**

monitoring
  equipment 36
  fluid therapy 111
  patient 31–6, 59–60
  postanaesthesia care unit 100–1
  potential hazards 59–60
  regional anaesthesia 84
  see also individual procedures
morphine **47, 115**
  see also opioids
motor block 118
multiple organ dysfunction syndrome (MODS) 144
musculoskeletal system, physical examination 6
myocardial infarction 3, 148–9
  non-ST-segment-elevation (NSTEMI) 148
  ST-segment-elevation (NSTEMI) 148–9, *148*

naloxone 113
nasal cannulae 104–5, *105*
nasopharyngeal airway 19, *19*, 64–5, *65*
National Confidential Enquiry into Perioperative
    Outcome and Death (NCEPOD) 13
nausea and vomiting
  central neural blockade 84–5
  postoperative (PONV) 50, 108, *109*
needle cricothyroidotomy *97*, 98
nervous system, physical examination 6
neuromuscular blocking drugs 44–6, **45**
  anticholinesterases 45–6
  assessment of blockade 74–5
  depolarizing 44–5
  non-depolarizing 45
  see also individual drugs
neuromuscular disorders 5
nitrous oxide 24–5, 42, 43
  cylinder colour **24**
  systemic effects 43
non-steroidal anti-inflammatory drugs *see* NSAIDs
NSAIDs 49
  contraindications **49**
nurses, preoperative assessment by 2

obese patients 10–11, **10, 11**
obstetric patients 89–91
  aortocaval compression 90–1
obstructive sleep apnoea 10–11
oesophageal Doppler cardiac output monitoring 34–5, *35*
oesophageal intubation, unrecognised 69
oesophageal speech 134
oliguria 106, 145–7
  investigations 146–7
omeprazole 40
ondansetron **50**, *109*
one-lung ventilation 91–2, *91*
opioids 46–9, **47**, 113, **115**
  central and peripheral effects **47**
  long-term complications 113
  narcosis 155

opioids (*Continued*)
  overdose   113
  pure agonists   46–8, **47**
  pure antagonists   48
  regulation of   48–9
  see also individual drugs
optical stylets   23, *23*
oral contraceptives   5
oropharyngeal (Guedel) airway   19, *19*, 63–4, *64*
oxygen   24
  alveolar concentration   **104**
  blood content   **104**
  cylinder colour   **24**
  inspired   **123**
    reduced concentration   104
  PaO_2 *102*, 128
  supply monitoring   36
oxygen delivery   104–6, *105*
  fixed-performance devices   105–6, *105*
  variable-performance devices   104–5, *105*
oxygen masks   104–5, *105*
oxygen saturation   **123**
$PaCO_2$ *102*, 128
PaO_2 *102*, 128
pain
  acute   112–13, **113**
  experience of   112
  and hypoxaemia   103
  difficult problems   119
  management *see* analgesia
pancuronium   **45**
paracetamol   40, 49
parecoxib   49
patient-controlled analgesia (PCA)   114–15
  advantages and disadvantages   115
patients
  acutely ill *see* acutely ill patients
  informed consent   14–15
  monitoring   31–6, 59–60
    see also individual procedures
  positioning   72–4
    lateral   73, *73*
    prone   73–4, *74*
    supine   72–3, *72*
  preoperative check   58–9
  sign in   59
  warming   30–1, 70
pericardial rub   128
peripheral nerve blocks   115–16
peripheral nerve stimulator   33
pethidine   **47**
physical examination
  acutely ill patients   130
  anaesthetic assessment   6–8
platelet concentrates   55
pneumonia   137
  investigations   137
  treatment   137

pneumothorax   103, 138
  investigations
  monitoring
  treatment
pollution   29–30
positive end-expiratory pressure (PEEP)   28
positive pressure ventilation   71–2
post dural puncture headache   85, 118–19
post-anaesthesia care   100–21
  analgesia   112–19
  complications *see* postoperative complications
  fluid therapy   108–11
postanaesthesia care unit   100–1
  discharge from   101, **101**
postoperative analgesia   113
postoperative complications   101–8
  hypertension   108
  hypotension   106–7
  hypoxaemia   101–4
postoperative nausea and vomiting (PONV)   50,
    108, *109*
pregnancy   6
premedication   39–40
  analgesia   40
  anti-emetics   40
  pH/volume of gastric contents   39–40
preoperative assessment
  anaesthetist-led   2–3
  baseline investigations   **2**
  investigations   2
  nurse-led   2
preoperative assessment clinic   2–3
preoperative checks   58–9
  anaesthetic machine   58
  patient   58–9
  sign in   59
preoxygenation   62
preparation for surgery   1–17
pressure controlled ventilation (PCV)   28
pressure support ventilation (PSV)   28
prilocaine   52
prochlorperazine   *109*
prone position   73–4, *74*
propofol   **41**
  total intravenous anaesthesia   70–1
pruritus   118
pseudocholinesterase deficiency   44–5
pulmonary diffusion defects   104
pulmonary embolism   140–1, *140*
  investigations
  treatment
pulmonary function tests   8
pulmonary oedema   139–40
  causes   **139**
  monitoring
  treatment
  investigations   139–40, *140*
pulse   **123**

pulse analysis cardiac output monitoring   35
PiCCO®
LiDCO®
Flotrac®
pulse oximetry   32, 127

ranitidine   40
rapid sequence induction   89
recreational drugs   6
red cell concentrates   55
regional anaesthesia   79–86
   awake vs. anaesthetised patients   86
   caesarean section   89–90
   monitoring   84
   postoperative   115–19, *116*
   role of   79–80
   techniques   80–4
     see also specific blocks
remifentanil   **47**
renal disease
   acute kidney injury   **145**
   medical referral   9
renal failure   5
   pre-renal vs. intrinsic   **146**
respiration rate   **123**
respiratory depression   117–18
respiratory disease
   medical referral   9–10
   signs of   127
   see also individual conditions
respiratory system
   history   4
   obese patients   10–11, **11**
   physical examination   6
rheumatoid disease   5
Ringer's lactate   54
risk indicators   12–13, **12**
rivaroxaban   14
rocuronium   **45**
ropivacaine   52, **53**

salbutamol   94
saltatory conduction   51
scavenging systems   29–30
Schedule 2 drugs
   supply and custody 48
Seldinger technique   61
Sellick's manoeuvre   89, *89*
sepsis/septic shock   143–4
   treatment   144
sevoflurane   **42**
shock
   cardiogenic   144–5
   hypovolaemic   84, 106, 142–3
   septic   143–4
sickle-cell screen (sickledex)   8
sign in   59

sign out   76–7
silent chest   134
sinus bradycardia   107
sinus tachycardia   107
Situation Background Assessment Recommendation
   (SBAR)   122
skin sepsis   84
smoking   5–6
social history   5–6
   smoking
   alcohol
   drugs
   pregnancy
sodium chloride 0.9%   **54**
sodium citrate, oral   40
spinal anaesthesia   83, *83*
   caesarean section   90
   contraindications   84
   postoperative   119
spontaneous ventilation   71, 76–7
status epilepticus   156
   treatment   156
   investigations   156
steroids   40, 94
stress response   111
stroke   155–6, *155*
   treatment   155
   CT scan   156
subclavian vein, cannulation   61
sugammadex   46
supine position   72–3, *72*
supraglottic airway devices   19–22, *20, 21,* 66–7, *66,* 76–7
   aspiration with   93
   insertion   66–7, *66*
operation, classification of   13
suxamethonium   44
   side effects   **44**
syringe pumps   31
systemic inflammatory response syndrome (SIRS)   143

tachycardias   149–50
   postoperative   107
target controlled infusion   70
temperature   **123**
   hypothermia   103
   malignant hyperpyrexia   95
   monitoring   33–4
   patient warming   30–1
tension pneumothorax   138
   treatment 138
thiopental   **41**
thoracotomy   91–2, *91*
thyromental distance   7, *8*
total intravenous anaesthesia (TIVA)   44
   advantages   71
   disadvantages   71
   maintenance   70–1

tracheal intubation 67–9
  complications 69
  confirmation of position 68–9
  difficult 95–6, *96*
  equipment 67
  failed 96, 98
  indications **67**
  reflex activity 69
  technique 67–8, *68*
  tracheal tubes 20–2, *21*
  tracheal tubes
    reinforced
    preformed
    double lumen
    uncuffed
tracheostomy, blocked 133–4, *135*
track and trigger systems 122–3, **123**
tramadol 47–8
transfer to operating theatre 72–4
  anaesthetic record 76
  assessment of neuromuscular blockade 74–5
  intraoperative fluids 75–6
  patient positioning 72–4, *72, 73*
  time out 74
transthoracic echocardiography 143
transversus abdominis plane block 81, *81*, 116
trauma during tracheal intubation 69
Trendelenburg position 73

ultrasound 31
unconscious patients 132
  coma 129–30
  Glasgow Coma Scale **130**
  hypoglycaemia 154–5

hypoxaemia/hypovolaemia 157
informed consent 16
opioid narcosis 155
status epilepticus 156
stroke/intracranial haemorrhage 155–6, *155*
urea 8
urinalysis 147
urinary retention 118
urine output
  absent *see* anuria
  low *see* oliguria

vacuum 25
vaporizers 26, *26*
vapour concentration analysis 33
vasodilatation 107
vecuronium **45**
venous thromboembolism, prevention 13–14
ventilation 100, 128
  impaired mechanics 102
  mechanical *see* mechanical ventilation
  modes of 28
  one-lung 91–2, *91*
  positive pressure 71–2
  spontaneous 71, 76–7
  see also breathing systems
ventilation-perfusion mismatch 103–4, **104**
videolaryngoscopes 23
Volulyte **55**
Voluven **55**
vomiting *see* nausea and vomiting

warming of patients 30–1, 70
Wilson score 7

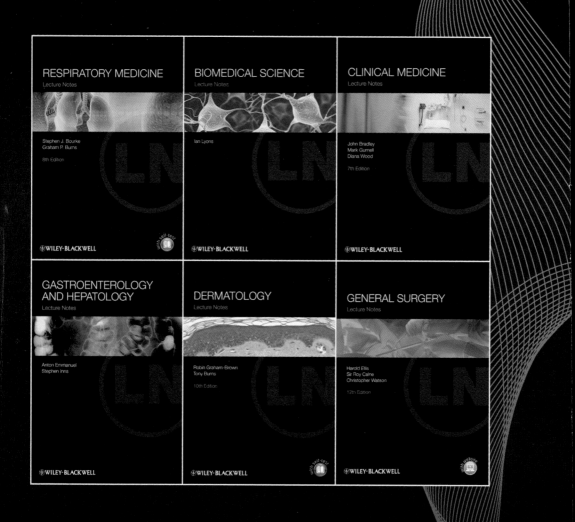
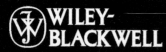